30 Days Fit Body Meal And Workout Plan

Table of Contents

Who I am? 1

Introduction 3

Macronutrients...6

Carbohydrates...10

Proteins 13

Fats..16

How to stop limiting yourself...........................19

What should always be in the fridge 22

Glycemic index..24

Water 27

Replace sugar...30

Supplements and sports nutrition 32

Diet disruptions..37

Public catering 39

Actual meal plan..41

Cellulite 44

Menstrual cycle...47

Training when not feeling well..........................49

Before and after workout meal 50

Warm up and stretching..................................52

Cardio 54

How to target a problem zone 56

Personal training program 57

Recovery 70

Motivation 72

Conclusion 75

Healthy recipe book 77

Who I am?

My name is Natalia Zorina and I've seen many personal trainers who look worse than their own clients and I was always wondering how someone would ever pay for their services. I would never hire a personal trainer who does not look like my dream body. I take a personal trainer as a motivation and an example of who I should become. Sure we all different and maybe your thinking is different. I know someone prefers to have a personal trainer who chats lots, someone pays attention to credentials and certifications. So let me introduce myself do you know who wrote this book.

In general words, I am a wife, mother, social media fitness blogger, personal trainer and since now a writer. I am also a fitness bikini athlete. Was lucky to step on stages both in Europe and North America.

Honestly speaking, I've created so many articles for my online audience during a couple of years, so all I had to do is to put all my articles together in one book.

How I got involved in fitness and social media? Here is a story. I am originally from eastern Europe and moved to New York when I was 18. Crazy life pace, lack of time and money made me eat unhealthy fast foods so I gained 12 kilograms in 3 months. As for a lady who was 50 kilograms before this trip, it was a big gain. I returned back home and decided to lose weight, but it was not as easy as I expected, so I started learning in order to help myself. I lost those kilograms and was ready to go back to North America, this time I was going to study in Toronto. I knew I can get in same trouble there, so I decided to keep this under control. I was working out, ate healthy foods and I went quite far. I got not just skinny, but sporty body and feeling of being absolutely healthy. At that time I decided that I also should share my knowledge with others, so I can help someone who needs motivation and directions. I got certification in nutrition and personal training. And till now my main desire is to help other become fit and healthy.

Introduction

From the very first time, when one of my friends asked me to help to get back into a good shape, I thought that I can write a meal and workout plan with no problem. But if I did that, then she would go back to what she is used to, right after finishing that meal plan. So that is why I wanted to not just give her a schedule and instructions of what to eat and how to workout, but also to teach her what is good and what is bad for health and body.

I knew it would take at least 4 months to reach her goal of losing 15 kilograms, and plus she needed not just lose weight, but also learn how to maintain at the desired level. So you want to know what I did? I haven't created any unique pill or invented unusual method of losing weight, I was just explaining to her a theory of the healthy lifestyle is a short and easy to understand manner, so she can learn and remember easily. After this "theory part" I planned to write that meal and workout plan, but guess what? My friend was able to do that herself now, without my help. This experience made me decide that this is the way I am going to go with all my future clients. Sure it is a lot easier to write that meal plan for 30 days as all other coaches do. And after selling a plan they usually are waiting for a client to come back for another, next month plan. But I am not a person who wants to make money in any possible way. I prefer to help people to learn these pretty easy health related topics. I prefer to make people's life better.

So this was a short introduction into why this book is not just a ready meal and workout plan, but a navigator in the most important information, which will help you to learn what to eat and how to workout. And I promise, no difficult terms.

This book is not what my clients usually get. This is something special, something that is going to work with every person. As I said, after reading this book you will not just have personal meal and workout plan, but also a knowledge that will let you move towards your dream body step by step.

You have this book in your hands means that you are a bit closer to your dream body already. You know, I've had a lot of clients, who bought meal plans, realized that it is a lot of work, changes and restrictions, and decided to never put that plan into action. But it is still ok, I am still proud of those people. You know why? Because they realized that they are willing to change. And I believe that one day they will be ready for action towards changes. We all different, and for some people, it makes take more time and more tries until things will more forward. So do not worry, you will change as much as you want, you can do it. All you have to do is to read all I wrote in this book and take this knowledge into a real life as soon as you can. With the dream body, you will also receive stronger health, power, and endurance.

My book is divided into 3 parts: nutrition, workout, and healthy recipes. I made a decision to give you 100 healthy recipes, so you can see that healthy foods can be also delicious and easy to cook. I am sure it will be helpful at the beginning, it will be your source of ideas. After that, you will be able to create your own. I am sure about it.

Why do I choose to combine both nutrition and workout information? Because they do not work separately. There is no sense to workout if you are not eating healthy. You will understand this in details, you will know what is good for your body.

Very important to remember that this book is not a magic tool to create you a new body, this is a source of knowledge that will help you to understand how to create that new body.

Ok, I am sure you cannot wait to start the process. Let's do it right now!

Macronutrients

Sporty body is built in the kitchen. I am sure you have heard this catchphrase. 80% of your success depends on nutrition. Therefore, the first thing we will deal with is nutrition. In this chapter, we will talk about the most important topics that will help you to learn how to eat in a balanced way.

You've probably heard that nutritionists recommend counting calories, proteins, fats and carbohydrates if you want to lose weight, but do you really need to adhere to numbers and diligently count calories, proteins, fats, and carbohydrates? My answer is: YES and NO.

Are you experiencing difficulties or ambiguity with the amount of foods to eat? Try to use an on-line calorie counter (for example MyFitnessPal) for a couple of days. It will make you understand whether you are overeating or not. After a while, you will be able to intuitively understand how much you need to eat and what exactly you need to eat.

When preparing your nutrition plan, pay attention to:

- caloric content and proportion of proteins, fats, and carbohydrates (chocolate bars have an equal amount of calories as a vegetable salad with fish or chicken, but they have a totally different effect on the quality of the body)

- regularity of meals (There is a huge difference between dividing 1500 kcal into 5 - 6 equal parts and consuming them all in one single heavy meal)

- variety (healthy foods can be tasty, there is no need to eat only spinach and chicken breast all day long)

- experiment (psychologically it is easier to stay away from unhealthy foods if your meals are different and unusual)

- rely on the result, not the scale. In fact, a formula is not the best way to correctly calculate the optimal number of calories, proteins, fats and carbohydrates. Only tests in the laboratory can tell what amount and proportion of macronutrients should be consumed. Tests show whether you have shortage or excess of macronutrients and micronutrients. Based on that, you will be advised on a diet plan. After implementing, you should do tests again and see how things change.

You probably still want to do calculations and find out how many calories and macronutrients your body needs, right? First of all, you should decide on your desired weight. But it should be not less than 6 kilograms that your weight right now. If it is less, then you should do redo calculation every 6 kilograms you lose.

Fats, proteins, and carbohydrates are macronutrients. Each gram of each contains a certain amount of calories:

- 1 gram of fat has 9 kcal

- 1 gram of proteins has 4 kcal

- 1 gram of carbohydrates has 4 kcal

How much does our body need each of the macronutrients?

Your body needs 0,8 - 1,2 grams of fat per each kilogram of the body weight. For example, if your weight is 50 kg you need about 40-60 grams of fat (which equals to 360-540 kcal).

Your body needs 1,5 - 2 grams of protein per each kilogram of the body weight. For example, if your weight is 50 kg you need about 75-100 grams of proteins (300-400 kcal).

You should have 3 - 5 grams of carbohydrates per each kilogram of the body weight. For example, if your weight is 50 kg you need about 150-250 grams (600-1000 kcal).

Now let's count how many calories should be consumed in 1 day if current body weight is 50 kilograms. 360+300+600=1260 - bottom calories point. 540+400+1000=1940 - top calories point. As you can see there is a quite difference between the bottom and top limits, so take the average value and see how your body reacts. After that, increase or decrease the calorie content depending on your goal - weight loss, weight gain or maintaining. But please remember, there should be no sudden weight increases, implement changes gradually. In case you are breastfeeding, please add another 300-500 kcal to the total caloric intake.

Now you have formula, but I propose to replace all calculations with a scheme that will help you understand how your menu should look like on everyday basis, It should consist of grains, fruits, chicken, milk products (yoghurt, cottage cheese, milk), fish, vegetables, nuts, coffee, tea, water. The size of meal portions and the choice of foods depends on such factors as your current weight, lifestyle, pace and schedule, and so on. Do not worry, we will talk about this in details later.

As you can see I did not need to devote a lot of time to this topic and this short scheme is proof that a rational, balanced diet is easy.

Carbohydrates

Let's make things clear! The most important thing you have to understand is that carbohydrates are necessary. It is popular now to cut carbs and start a fat cutting process. People choose this strategy without really finding out details about it, but I can tell you already that small intake of carbohydrates is the big mistake you can do.

Carbohydrates can be conventionally divided into 3 types: sugar, starch, and fiber.

Starches (also known as complex carbohydrates) are oats, barley, rice, vegetables like corn, potatoes, beans, corn, rye, buckwheat, kinda, etc. These foods give us long-term energy, but how does it all work and why they are called complex? Here is what happen after you eat a cup of barley. Your body starts to break down complex carbohydrate into simple. It works by extracting protein, amino acids and other useful substances from that barley. Gradual splitting up to glucose occurs. Glucose gradually gives energy to the brain, muscles and your whole body. As a result, you feel fed for several hours. Starches are great for people who choose a healthy lifestyle and watching the weight. You can eat them for breakfast, for example, and won't be hungry until the next meal. You won't have any problems with those accident unhealthy snacks in the middle of the day because now you feel full until another healthy meal.

Sugars (simple or fast-acting carbohydrate) are cakes, ice cream, sweets, milk chocolate, jam, honey, soft drinks, packaged juices, syrups, fruits, etc. Sucrose, fructose, lactose are also fast-acting carbohydrates. They are called fast-acting because they are breaking down and digesting very fast. This means that they give energy to your body very soon after you eat them. That is why they will give you a feeling satisfaction and will make you full for not more than one hour. Let's look at it as if it was a circle. You eat the cake > blood sugar level goes up > insulin level goes up > insulin turns this sugar into storage (fat) > food you ate is fully digested and source of energy is empty > sugar level drops sharply > you begin feeling hungry > your brain gives a signal that it requires another dose of simple carbohydrates > you eat the cake again. This "circle" is really the number one reason why people have excessive weight.

Fiber is part of vegetables, legumes, bran, fruits, nuts, seeds. Fiber does not exist in the animal products because it comes from plant foods. Fiber slows down the digestion of carbohydrates, proteins, and fats. It also contributes to digestive health. You feel full and satisfied after eating fibers, so it can be helpful for weight loss. For good health, adults need to try to eat 25 to 30 grams of fiber each day. Fiber increases a volume of foods you eat, means you feel more satisfied even though you eat the same amount of foods. It also reduces appetite, increases the absorption of nutrients, minerals, vitamins and essential fatty acids.

Based on the information above, you need to eat starches during the day, 1-2 fruits and at least 300 grams of vegetables per day. In addition to that, add nuts or dried seeds to your meals.

Proteins

Proteins are the basis of life. Also, it is one of the basic elements of our nutrition and a part of all cells in our body. Our muscles, organs, skin and hair consist of protein.

Let's find out why we all need protein and in what cases it can bring harm to our bodies. Proteins are high molecular organic substances consisting of amino acids. They are complex molecules that are capable of entering into complex interactions. Let me explain in simple words, they are such "bricks", with a wide range of possibilities, so they can be both building material, a carrier of other substances, and conductor of complex chemical reactions. As I said before, protein itself consists of amino acids. There are 21 kinds of amino acids, but 8 of them (valine, isoleucine, leucine, lysine, methionine, threonine, tryptophan and phenylalanine) are vital for humans and therefore they are called essential amino acids. This means that human body cannot synthesize (produce) them itself. So these 8 amino acids must come from food.

There is a wide range of functions that proteins perform. First one is "protection": proteins support the immune system. Antibodies that protect us from infections and viruses are immunoglobulin proteins. Second is "regulation": proteins produce various elements that are necessary for proper functioning of human body. For example, hemoglobin, enzymes, gastric juice, vitamins. Third, "structural": our hair and nails consist of collagen protein, our muscles consist mainly of myosin and actin proteins. Forth, "transportation": erythrocytes (red blood cells) are made of proteins and lipids and are part of the cardiovascular system, which provides transportation of nutrients, oxygen, carbon dioxide, hormones, and blood cells to and from the cells in the body. Also, hemoglobin is a transport protein that carries oxygen and carbon dioxide. Fifth protein function is "energy function": as I said earlier there are 4 calories in each gram of protein, which our body can use as an energy source. Why do I tell you all this? Because I want you to realize how important it is to provide enough protein to your body.

Proteins are a good source of energy, but it is used only after carbohydrates and fats are depleted as energy sources. What I mean is that human body uses energy from carbohydrates and fats first, and only then starts to use proteins.

Animal proteins have better-balanced composition of essential amino acids than vegetable origin. In this regard, the diet of vegetarians turns out to be much poorer and requires careful consideration in order to obtain necessary substances. Sources of animal protein: dairy, meat, fish and eggs.

Plant proteins also contain essential amino acids, however not as much as in animal proteins. Sources of vegetable protein are soy, nuts, legumes (lentils, peas, beans), cereals, whole grains.

Recommended daily protein dose is 0,84 grams per each kilogram of body weight (according to the World Health Organization). People who have an active lifestyle (weight lifting, running, yoga, etc) need about 1-1,8 grams of protein per each kilogram of the body weight, due to a necessity to increase its' synthesis in muscle fibers.

Protein really plays a very important role in our body. Nobody can be healthy if there is a weak protein consumption. However, excessive intake of protein is also associated with health risks. According to the studies, excessive consumption of animal protein increases the risk of kidney stones by 250%. Moreover, excessive protein intake may be associated with the development of osteoporosis (bone weakness increases the risk of a broken bone). So if you have related health problems, I advise being consulted by the doctor before you choose a high-protein diet.

Fats

Are you still stay away from fats because you think they are dangerous for your fit body? Let's look at it in details. Usually, individual who decided to lose weight starts to immediately avoid products with a high-fat content. But there is a surprising mistake in such decision. Reduction of fat, on the contrary, prevents from losing weight and is very harmful to our health, especially for females!

Why? First of all, your brain needs fats. It is like a shield for our brain and it protects its' membranes. This means that your brain activity will suffer from fats intake reduction.

Secondly, fat is a great source of energy. You are right, the primary and main energy source is carbohydrates, but fat is an alternative power for our body.

Third reason is that fat gives us a feeling of being full and satisfied. If you are following low-fat diet your sense of satiety will be extremely short. Fat releases a hormone that regulates that food shifting speed from the stomach into the intestine. As a result, we are fed longer and we need less food.

The fourth reason, fats do not increase blood sugar. That's why it's better to eat a piece of dark chocolate instead of milk chocolate bar. From such treat, there will be no harm.

Fifth reason, fat promotes vitamins. Salad with olive oil is better than a salad with low-fat dressing, because part of the vitamins from the food are fat-soluble, which means that they need fats for their assimilation. For the same reason, it is not advised to eat fat-free cottage cheese. But you can always add some almond butter, nuts or coconut chips to fat-free cottage cheese, to made it delicious and vitamin-rich.

So now you know why your body needs fats, but there are different kinds of fats and now I am going to tell you which ones you need and which ones you should avoid. Generally speaking, there are useful and not useful fats.

Saturated fat stays solid even at room temperature. For example, they are in red meat and milk. This type of fat increases the "bad" cholesterol in the body and increases the risk of cardiovascular disease. The safe zone is to keep up to 10% of daily calories coming from saturated fats. For example, if you consume 1800 calories, then you should eat up to 180 calories from saturated fat, which is about 20 grams.

Trans-unsaturated fatty acids. You better stay away from these guys. Trans fat is a synthetic product. It means that it is produced and added to products artificially. You ask me why they add it to foods if they are bad for health? The answer is very easy. They add it trans fats make products last longer (longer expiration date) and they make it cheaper to produce. Eating trans fat is really the worst thing we can do with our health and longevity. Such fats not only increase "bad" cholesterol but also reduce the content of "good" cholesterol in the blood. Please eat 0 grams of trans fats per day.

Saturated and polyunsaturated fats. These fats are considered to be healthy fats. You can find them is such foods as almonds, cashew, walnut, peanut, cheese, yogurt, dark chocolate, avocado. Omega-3 fatty acid contains in flax seeds, chia seeds, walnuts, salmon, tofu, sardines, etc. Even healthy fats need an adequate approach. When losing weight, keep a fat balance of 30-40% animal fat and 60-70% plant fat. When the goal is achieved, change proportion to 50/50 or 60/40. Regardless of the goals (weight loss, maintenance) - the optimal amount of fats per day is 0,8-1,2 grams per each kilogram of your desired weight. You should try various proportions and amounts until you find your own perfect balance.

How to stop limiting yourself

Proper healthy nutrition often associated with a lot of restrictions, but it's not entirely true. Usually, only beginners have this association, but experienced healthy lifestylers can easily explain that it is not true. It is all about making balanced nutrition your habit, rather than limited in time life goal. It is not about making you stay away from treats until the end of your life. There is no need to abandon desired (even if it's a chocolate bar), but you should learn how to feel an adequate amount of desired. Means, 10 chocolate bars at a time is not good. Lots of people cannot control proper number, amount, and frequency of meals. They fail diet soon and overeat instead. I am sure you've experienced this at least once. In this chapter, I offer you two ideas of how not to fail new meal plan. Both methods are based primarily on psychology, in order to exclude failures smoothly and with no stress:

Method #1 is based on the theory of accessibility of the desired (or minimizing effort). What does it mean? This means that something that you want to eliminate from your life should become inaccessible. For example, if you are willing to eliminate chocolate muffins, then you should not bring them home from the store, and every time you want to eat a muffin, you will need to make an effort and go to that store. If you still decide to make that effort, buy only one muffin and go home, so each muffin will cost you a trip to the store. Sure this won't work if you will keep walking back and forward all day long, but this will save you from eating them before bed for sure because the store is closed at night and you have none available at home. In other words, you have to make a big effort and overcome a specific path in order to get that desired piece. Conversely, if you decide to eat more vegetables or drink more water, it should always be at home and stand handy. For example, wash vegetables and place them in the bowl right next to you, so you do not need to make any effort to reach them at any time. Carry that water bottle with you around the house, put it in the bag when going outside. And after a while, you will see that this become your habit, good habit.

My friend, famous dancer told me about this theory. But her example was not about vegetables or water. She wanted to start early morning runs, so she went to bed in a t-shirt and kept sneakers right next to the bed. Guess what? It took 15 seconds to dress up and be ready to run. This way there was no need to overcome any obstacles or make any effort. What I am trying to say is that this method can help you with almost anything.

Method #2 - cheat meal. I know in some families it is impossible not to bring those chocolate muffins at home because other family members do not want to eliminate them from their lives. And this is fair of course. So in this case I offer you to choose one day of the week when you will be allowed to have those desired but forbidden treats. For example, on Saturday you can have anything. But only one piece, not a whole store, deal? This way you will know that you can afford it, but just have to wait a little bit and that desired is waiting for you on Saturday.

What should always be in the fridge

It is quite obvious, that if you bring that cheeseburger, frozen pizza or carrot cake home, then sooner or later someone will eat them. You buy those cookies for a reason, right? As we discussed earlier, the best option is not to bring home what you want to eliminate from your diet. However, as I said before, most likely not all family members are willing to stop eating marshmallows along with you, so it is important to always have a "healthy snack" in the fridge in order to have something to eat when there is an irresistible desire to eat something or when there is not enough time for a proper meal.

So here is a list of healthy snacks ideas:

- Portioned walnut paste or mix of nuts (tasty, nutritious, healthy)

- Frozen grapes (it does not become hard as a stone like other fruits and berries, but make sure you not overeat them, because they are pretty high in sugar)

- Peas, green beans (crunchy and always ready to eat)

- Celery (it is ideal safe snack, because it is 95% made of water. It is really delicious with hummus)

- Carrots with hummus

- Tomato juice (make sure you buy 100% vegetable juice with a small amount of salt)
- Hard boiled eggs
- Dark chocolate

Glycemic index

Have you heard of glycemic index? This chapter will discuss what is a glycemic index, what do you need it for and whether you should take it into consideration or not.

Any carbohydrate entering the body can be used as an energy source only after it is processed to the simple component - glucose.

As you already know from the chapter about carbohydrates, some of them raise blood sugar rapidly, because they are able to break down to glucose very easily and fast (for example, white sugar or wheat bread). The glycemic index determines the effect of carbohydrate on blood sugar level. And it helps us to understand how quickly your body turns carbohydrates into glucose.

You may be wondering why should you care about sugar, insulin and glycemic index.

Some food gives out a very large amount of energy right away, as soon as it was chewed, and the other can give us even more energy, but gradually during a long period of time. In the first case, insulin comes into a play immediately. Insulin lowers the level of sugar in the blood and contributes so your body begins to store energy creating fat. If energy is given gradually and by small portions, there will be no high rise of sugar, so insulin will not put glucose in reserve. As a result, insulin will not contribute to the formation of the fatty layer.

So it turns out that it is not about calories, but about even low high-calorie product can increase the waist, and high-calorie - to promote weight loss.

The smaller the glycemic index, the less the influence it has on a blood sugar raise:

- 55 or less - low (good)
- 56-69 - medium
- 70 and more - high (bad)

A low value indicates that the product practically does not cause fluctuations in the levels of sugar and insulin in the blood. The average value causes a moderate increase in glucose levels. Products with low and medium glycemic indexes are preferable in the food pyramid.

Glycemic index table of all products is available on the Internet, but they can vary. And it depends on the process of cooking, or rather - the way products are processed.

Remember, the fewer fibers in food, the higher glycemic index.

But, products with high glycemic index are not always bad. Here is why. When they talk about glycemic index, we usually forget about the fact that there is also a glycemic load - the amount of carbohydrates in a dose (unit volume). The high glycemic index does not always mean that this food should be excluded. For example, watermelon has a glycemic index equal to 72, which is really high, but its' glycemic load is 4 grams of carbohydrates per each 100 grams of watermelon, which is an extremely low indicator. So an analysis of these two indicators speaks of the "goodness" of certain foods in the human diet.

Why is glycemic index important? In addition to influencing body shape, foods with low glycemic index are associated with a reduction of the risk of heart disease, type 2 diabetes, metabolic syndrome, stroke, depression, chronic kidney disease, gallstones, neural tube defects, uterine fibroids and such types of cancers as breast, colon, prostate and pancreas.

Water

Water consumption is very important. It is not less important that protein, fats and carbohydrates intake.

I am sure you've heard how much water you should drink, but let us repeat everything so it is clarified. You should drink not less than 2 liters of pure drinking water per day. It should be divided into portions throughout the day. For self-control, pour water into a 2 liters bottle and finish it during the day. Drink when you want, except during having your meal. Keep drinking pure water during training (especially cardio), at least 0,5 liters during one session.

Coffee. Sure you can drink coffee, choose natural ground coffee. 2-3 cups of coffee a day is completely fine if you feel good after them and have no problems with the heart. It is also fine to have a little milk and even sugar. But do not go crazy and put 3 spoons of sugar and cream instead of milk, ok? Learn to appreciate the real taste of coffee! Coffee is not instead pure water. Coffee goes separately. You still should drink 2 liters of pure water. Moreover, for each cup of coffee, you should drink an extra glass of pure water.

Tea. If it is green or black tea, then it is similar to what I said about coffee.

Soup. You will be surprised but many people think that soup can be count as water. This is not right. It is liquid, but not water. Soup is a meal and you should add it to your daily calorie count.

Juice. Forget about packed juice from the store. No matter what they write on the label, it is artificial and fully packed with sugar and chemicals. Freshly squeezed juice is a great choice, but also should be added to the daily calorie count.

Alcohol. One glass of red or white dry wine is what you should choose with your dinner one-twice a week. Beer is the worst thing you can do for your waist. Cocktails are packed with empty calories which will be stored in cellulite right away.

Soft drinks. I know quite a lot of people who switched to a healthy lifestyle, excluded sugars but start drinking those sweet sodas with a confidence that it would not hurt the progress. They like to have those sweet drinks because it satisfies their cravings for sweets. Let's see what they are made of and how they affect your body and health in general. To be honest, there are hundreds of reasons why you should not drink them, and I would need to write a whole book in order to talk about every reason. Soft drink is an explosive mixture of phosphoric acid, sugar, caffeine, artificial colors and flavors. I guarantee you that you will get faster results in slimming, getting rid of cellulite and gaining toned skin if you stop drinking soft drinks.

Zero sugar drinks are not any better. They are not dietary products. There are 2 most popular sweetness in zero sugar drinks: aspartame -

synthetic sweetener, it includes phenylalanine which depletes the stores of serotonin (a hormone of joy), which leads to depression, anger, panic, violence. Saccharin is another artificial sweetener, it has no calories, while 300-500 times sweeter than table sugar. It seems that everything is fine with it, but it accumulates in the bladder and genital organs and activates cancer cells. Do you want some more or this is enough to stop killing yourself with those soft drinks?

Conclusion: drink enough water, and treat yourself with a quality natural coffee and tea.

Replace sugar

I just said all these terrible things about sugars and sweetness, so you probably decided to stay away from them. You are right white sugar and sweetness are useless and unhealthy, but it does not mean that we should stop treating ourselves with sweet foods. Let's look at how you ca replace sugar.

First, let me tell you what should not become a substitute for sugar:

- Honey, maple syrup and similar. They are healthy, but they have exactly the same amount of calories and causing same high glucose rise in the blood as table sugar does.

- Cane Sugar. It is absolutely useless to replace one similar product with the other. Moreover, often cane sugar is tinted white sugar.

- Chemical sweeteners. There are many side effects caused by chemical sweetness, but sure manufacturers do not want to mention them. The safest is Sucralose.

- Fructose. It has low glycemic index, so it deserved to be called a dietary product. However, some impressive researchers published data that fructose increases the rate of fat formation in humans.

- Stevia. It is extracted from the leaves of the plant species Stevia. It has a special taste but has a very natural origin. It does not cause a rise of insulin and can be used in cooking.

And now I will tell you about what can become a substitute for sugar. I am talking about healthy natural homemade sweets. This is the best option! For example, baked pears and apples, dietary oatmeal cookies, cottage cheese casserole, protein pancakes. In the end of this book, you will find lots of recipes you can try.

I know this is not what you wanted to hear, but this is true. There is no way to eat those cakes and lose weight. You should start watching what you eat right now.

Some of you may argue that sugar is needed for brain work. So I decided to prepare an answer right away. The human brain needs glucose, not sugar. But it is better to get it from complex carbohydrates (brown rice, vegetables).

Supplements and sports nutrition

I am sure you bought at least one pack of vitamins in your life. Have you heard that it is recommended to use a complex of vitamins and minerals to maintain the muscles of the joints, bones, Nervous, and cardiovascular systems when doing sports?

Drug stores offer such a huge selection of food additives, sports nutrition products, and vitamin complexes nowadays. Those companies develop attractive packaging, they are very bright and it makes us want to buy literally everything. Moreover, lots of people get the impression that there will be no result without these special products.

What to look for and how to choose what you really need? If we are not talking about bodybuilding competition preparation. then all you really need is a quality multivitamin. You will be surprised, but it is not very important how big is the amount of vitamins and minerals in your vitamin complex because your body is able to absorb limited volume and this volume is different for each individual. Your body will absorb as much as it needs at the moment. Therefore, I recommend paying attention to the quality of the vitamin complex. I recommend two multivitamins to choose from: Opti-Men/women Multivitamin (produced by Optimum Nutrition) or RAW One (Produced by Garden of Life). Both complexes performed well. I have been taking them for many years myself and offered my clients.

Perhaps you also want to know whether it worth buying a fat burner, protein, L-carnitine? Here is some information about this.

Protein powder is unnecessary if your protein intake is at a proper level. A powder is a substitute, it is not any better that eating proper protein meal. A portion of pure protein powder (usually 40 grams of protein in 1 scoop) can be replaced by egg whites, low-fat cheese, or chicken breasts without skin. It is common to take protein right after the strength training to make up the protein deficit so that muscles do not starve between the training session and your next full meal. If this is the case and you cannot have a meal soon after training, then you should try protein drinks. Therefore, you can always eat some of the above products instead of protein shake. It is also very convenient to drink a protein shake before cardio, for example. If you have no time to eat a good meal before training, then it might be not a good idea to workout, but you can always have some protein shake instead of a meal. Feed yourself with protein, so you have energy and strength during the training session.

So now you know that protein powder is not a panacea. It does not help to lose weight, gain muscles or anything else. It is just something convenient to use to replace regular meals. What matters is only your meal plan and time of consumption of certain foods. Protein powder is a well balanced composition of amino acids, it is very quickly absorbed, and it is a better choice than skipping a meal. But sure you can have results without it.

Fat burner stimulates metabolism in the body, suppresses appetite, reduces absorption of fats and carbohydrates from the digestive tract, blocks fat synthesis in adipose tissue and removes excess fluid. Mainly, fat burners accelerate the cleavage of fat molecules and convert fat into free energy, increasing its consumption. All this sounds beautiful and promising, but this will not happen if the consumer does not have a perfect diet and regular productive physical activities. Fat burners significantly affect nervous and cardiovascular systems, cause over-excitability, anxiety, insomnia, and it turns out that they have more minuses than pluses. It is much more effective and safer to concentrate on balanced nutrition and regular exercise.

Omega 3-6-9. First of all, remember, omega 9 is not essential fatty acids because our body is capable of producing it, so there is no need to take such supplements. Average person's nutrition habits cause an imbalance between omega 3 and omega 6. Why so? Let me explain. Omega 6 is found in a large number of different foods. For example, corn oil, nuts, soybean oil, sesame oil, margarine, chicken and meat fat, eggs, olives, avocado, dairy products. Omega 3 is not like that, it is contained in sea foods, fish and quite a bit in the chicken. From this, we can conclude that we consume a very small amount of omega 3 fatty acids. Perfectly, the ratio of these two fatty acids should be 1:1, well, or at least 5:1. Imbalance leads to fatigue problems with memory, overweight, dry skin, bad mood, circulatory disorders. From all of the above, we can conclude that we need to consume omega 3 as a dietary supplement, and I recommend Now Foods Omega 3 produced by Now Foods.

The last thing I want to talk about in this section is aloe vera juice. I received this kind of product for promotional purposes a while ago, I used it for about a year and I want to say that it was a successful experiment. I won't name the brand, so it does not look like a prophet them in my book, but I am sure you can find many quality products of this type on the market. This is an excellent addition to proper nutrition and a complex of vitamins. Here are 7 reasons to include Aloe in your diet:

1. Young and healthy skin. Our skin is being renewed every 3-4 weeks. Valuable substances that are part of the drinking aloe gel, help the skin fight the signs of aging and contribute to the emergence of new healthy cells.

2. Weight control. Regular use of aloe helps your body to naturally get rid of toxins, ensures the normal functioning of the digestive system and good metabolism, and this, in turn, pop up your energy level and helps to maintain a healthy weight.

3. Good digestion. A healthy digestive system ensures the ingestion of nutrients from the food we eat, into the blood, where they bring the maximum benefit to our body. Daily intake of aloe improves intestinal motility and promotes the growth of beneficial bacteria, thereby stimulating the penetration of nutrients into the blood.

4. Source of minerals. No matter how healthy your food may be, there may be a lack of minerals in it. Aloe contains minerals such as sodium, iron, potassium, chromium, magnesium, manganese, copper and zinc, etc.

5. The source of vitamins. Aloe contains a large number of vitamins that the body needs every day: A, B1, B2, B3, and B6, as well as vitamin E.

6. The source of essential amino acids. Amino acids are unique building blocks of our body as you already know. The composition of aloe products usually includes 8 amino acids, which are called irreplaceable and can not be produced by the body independently.

7. Strengthening the immune system. No good immune system means no resistance to diseases. Aloe with natural immune-fortifying substances will provide your immunity with natural support and effective protection.

Diet disruptions

What I mean by diet disruptions is when you cannot resist that craving and go off track. In this chapter, I will share some ideas about how to stay on track with joy.

Usually, new lifestyle starts very positively. You start reading some materials, getting motivated, start eating healthy food and workout. But at the same time, people and circumstances around you remain the same. They still eat that pasta under a thick layer of fatty cheese following by chocolate cake. And at some point of time, you start to have cravings. Please remember that you will have those cravings forever and never will get used to a healthy lifestyle if in your mind healthy foods mean "limitations" and unhealthy food means "freedom". Do you understand what I mean? I am sorry for being straight and tell you the truth as it is, but I believe you are enough adult to hear this. You should stop perceiving proper nutrition as a system of prohibitions. As long as you think so, your "healthy lifestyle" will be your temporary diet that you maintain for some time, but will go off sooner or later.

So here are some advices to follow:

- Stop dividing foods to the "right" and "wrong". You should not consider yourself as "good" if you eat well and "bad" if ate not what is planned.

- Understand what is proper nutrition. After this, you will feel those borders you cannot cross. But you can eat delicious meals that meet those requirements. Proper nutrition is not about chicken breast all day long.

- Keep in mind that first of all clean food is a contribution to your HEALTH.

- Understand that if you want you can always go back to your past life, eat sweet, fast food, alcohol, have bulging belly and cellulite.

Public catering

How to behave properly in public catering when you switched to clean eating? And how not to strain the situation with others who impose a cake, bread, and crackers with beer? My clients often ask me what to say to those friends and family members who just try to feed you no matter what. So here are a couple of advices:

- To have no meal is not an option! You are likely to be overwhelmed with questions and persuasions

- In fact, almost every café has one or more clean healthy choice in the menu. For example: salads, seafood, fresh squeezed juice or tea.

- Do not try to explain all the rules of healthy cooking to a waiter. They will ignore your request and cook as usual anyways, but your behavior will attract attention and cause questions from people you are meeting in the cafe

- If all they have in the menu is french fries and fatty dressings salads, then there is still a way to escape from that. Tell them you have stomach problem today, not feeling well and cannot have any meal. This always works for me!

- Remember what I said about alcohol before? Dry wine - yes. Strong spirits - no! First of all, this is not feminine, secondly, there are too many empty calories in it, and thirdly you will lose vigilance to what you eat, do and say.

Actual meal plan

Ok, it is time to finally create 30 days meal plan. Highlights:

- It is necessary to eat 5-6 times a day

- It is necessary to prepare and pack food in food containers for the whole day in advance, or even for a few days in advance

- Sweet (sugar, honey, desserts, fruits) should be excluded up to 20% of your food intake

- You should drink enough water as discussed earlier

So let's make things clear once again. First, you should calculate how many calories you need to consume based on your current weight minus 6 kilograms. For example, if your current weight is 80 kilograms, then you calculate how many calories you need per day using 74 kilograms. If you need to look up formulas again, go to the first chapter. Redo calculations each week. After you know how many calories you have, please use an application like MyFitnessPal (you can find it on-line) and insert your meals at least for a future couple of days. Add them to the application before you cook or eat them.

What foods can you add to your meal plan? You find a list of foods and beverages that can be used down below.

Vegetables: Broccoli, cauliflower, white cabbage, asparagus, greens (celery sprigs, parsley, dill, spinach), all kinds of deciduous lettuce, mushrooms, zucchini, eggplant, pumpkin, cucumbers, onion, green beans, bell pepper, radish, carrots, beets, avocados (make sure it fits daily fat consumption level), tomatoes, sweet potatoes etc.

Cooking method: fresh / boiled / grilled / in a double boiler / in a frying pan WITHOUT OIL! Very little auld should be added.

Drinks: pure water, green, red or black tea, coffee without milk (or with skimmed milk), herbal teas. Very little sugar can be added or should be replaced with stevia.

Protein foods: eggs, lean beef, veal, liver, chicken breasts (skinless), chicken hearts, lean ground chicken, turkey (breasts without skin), low fat cottage cheese (5% fat maximum), natural yogurt (low-fat), kefir (low-fat), low fat cheese (up to 20% fat), all variety of fish and seafood (shrimps, mussels, squid, scallops, real crab meat, octopus, etc.)

Cooking method: boil, grill, cook in a pan without oil, steam, bake. Little salt should be added. No canned food.

Carbohydrate foods: buckwheat, oatmeal, green peas, lentils, kidney beans, brown rice, long-grain rice, bulgur, couscous, quinoa, whole grain pasta, wholegrain bread, wholegrain crispy bread, rice bread with no added flavor, bran, etc.

You can add salt and organic spices, but to ready sauces should be added. All those dressings and sauces you find in stores are packed with sugar and chemicals. Please cook sauces yourself or go do organic stores like whole foods and find quality dressings.

How can you replace dressings? You can use soy sauce (not more than 1 tbsp per day), balsamic vinegar, olive oil, coconut oil.

You are all set, please go ahead and create that meal plan now.

Cellulite

Cellulite means structural changes in the subcutaneous fat layer, leading to a decrease of microcirculation and lymphatic outflow. There are different stages of cellulite. The first stage is when the "defect" is visible only at compression of a skin. But this is the norm for most women. A woman should maintain a subcutaneous fat layer at a rate of 15-25 percent in order to save her natural ability to have a baby. Otherwise, she will have problems with hormones, reproductive system, libido, kidneys and health in general.

Some women can get rid of cellulite completely, only when critically decrease weight, but this is very unhealthy and can be dangerous for health and life. If cellulite is obvious (stage 2-4) and brings discomfort, then you should take an action. Normally it is hard to get rid of cellulite because skin supply function is disrupted, and it is difficult to mobilize fat because of the lack of transport blood. If the blood supply is working well, then there should be sufficient physical activity to activate the process.

Now let's talk about causes of cellulite:

1. Genetics. The structure of the subcutaneous fat layer and the place of local accumulation of fat (fat depot) largely determine the degree of this skin problem.

2. Cooking. Unhealthy diet: low-carbohydrate or low-fat, or vice versa, use of food processed foods (refined sugar, salt, fatty, roasted, etc.) affects health and quality of the skin.

3. Not enough water consumption. Blood and lymph serve as a transport system. The thicker the blood, the harder it is to perform these functions. Water consumption regulates thickness.

4. Lack of physical activity. Contraction of muscles is a kind of "massage" for capillaries.

5. Low blood circulation (including a habit to cross legs when sitting).

6. Hormonal imbalance

7. Diseases of the digestive system, cardiovascular system, reproductive system.

Now you know reasons that can cause cellulite and probably wonder how to avoid this problem or how to get rid of it? Sure, here are top advises on this matter:

1. Drink a sufficient amount of water. Approximately 2 liters per day.

2. Integrate physical activity into your lifestyle. Muscle contractions contribute to a better outflow of blood and lymph. If there is no way to go to the gym - train at home or have a walk, run.

3. Contrast shower (alternate hot and cold water) has an effect on the skin condition and improves blood circulation.

4. Special body lotions and skin wraps that promote skin tone and elasticity. These will be useless if you do not establish a healthy, balanced eating habits. Watch for the intake of a sufficient amount of protein (about 1-2 grams of protein per each kilogram of your body). Avoid bad habits (smoking and alcohol).

To conclude, I would like to say that there will no miracle happen in one week. You need to approach the problem in a comprehensive manner. It is useless to expect any change if you are having nachos with beer before bed.

Menstrual cycle

We will now talk about the topic of the menstrual cycle, training, and nutrition. Most women think that only the period of menstruation requires attention, but there are several more phases that require not just your attention, but they also influence the result.

Phase 1: menstruation (1-5 day cycle). What happens to you: improved flexibility, reduced stamina, reduced muscle strength and reaction speed. What to do: replace strength training with stretching. If menstruation is especially painful, then you can generally have a day off. Nutrition: drink more liquid than usual, fewer carbohydrates, more easy to digest food.

Phase 2: follicular (6-13 day cycle). What happens to you: improved working capacity, endurance, readiness to work on all groups of muscles, and on the development of speed, endurance, and strength, metabolism is accelerated. What to do: this is the most productive phase, so there is no way to be lazy, do your best during the training session. Nutrition: accelerated metabolism allows you to consume more calories, but do not relax too much and you still should choose clean meals only. Add more carbohydrates after training.

Phase 3: ovulation (14-15 day cycle). What happens to you: the level of hormones at the maximum level. What to do: Continue training as in the previous phase, but it is advisable to add more flexibility exercises. In this phase, the biggest strengths results can be seen, so if you wanted to try heavy dumbbells - then this is the best time. Nutrition: you may feel hungry in this phase because of the acceleration of metabolism and it's good, eliminating hunger should be done through a balanced composition of proteins, carbohydrates, and fats.

Phase 4: luteal (16-28 day cycle). What happens to you: the metabolism slows down, so do not right the alarm if the weight increases slightly. In this period, you should not expect weight loss. What to do: during this period it is better to choose very energy-consuming types of fitness in order to compensate slow metabolism. Nutrition: more protein, fewer carbohydrates.

Training when not feeling well

Can I train with the flu? When to start training after recovery? Let's figure it out. For many of you who have just stepped on the path of self-improvement, flu is a big bummer. I know how it feels. You finally started a healthy lifestyle, you do everything correctly, you train, you go firmly to the goal, and then ["bang"] and you got sick. It feels really bad. And it should be noted that such a bummer happens quite often with beginners. Firstly, training for a beginner who has never done anything regularly before is always stressful. And the body can respond to it with a cold. Secondly, after training, sweaty and hot, many of you open the windows or stand under the air conditioner to cool down. Not the best things to do, right? As a result, you are sick and not sure whether you should keep training? Here is the answer:

1. It is better not to train even with the slightest signs of a cold. You should let the body recover

2. Let the situation go. Release those pessimistic thoughts. Yes, there will not be any planned workouts, but if you continue eating properly, then your body will be healthy again very soon

3. The first day without high body temperature, without symptoms of a cold is not a reason to immediately jump into equipment and start training. It is necessary to wait at least another two days after you feel cheerful and healthy.

Before and after workout meal

You should eat certain foods before and after your workout to make sure you have a proper supply during and after training. If you won't follow this, then you may have slow results. Please follow my instructions for better results.

Before workout:

- Eat at least 2 hours before your training session

- Eat a meal with proteins (lean meat/fish, dairy products, legumes) and complex carbohydrates (cereals, whole grain bread, etc).

- If you have less than an hour left before training, you still need to eat. Choose a small portion (100-200kcal) and it should be something that is quickly digested. For example, fruit, protein shake, protein bar, fruit smoothie.

- It's a myth that if you do not eat before training then there will be a calorie deficit and more fat will burn.

- Avoid fatty foods before exercise, they cause discomfort in the abdomen.

- If you do not eat before the beginning of the training, then you can not achieve a high level of intensity, because the body can not produce the right amount of energy.

- If you take a large amount of food or eat right before training, then during training your energy will be directed to food processing and not muscle work.

After workout:

- Post workout meal must contain both proteins and carbohydrates

- Caloric intake should be equal to half of the calories burned during the training session.

- Eat in 20-30 minutes after strength training or 30-60 minutes after aerobic training.

- You can drink in unlimited quantities (pure water).

Warm up and stretching

Very soon you will get to a chapter with your workout plan. Before that, I want to talk about the warm-up and its significance. Remember, a warm-up is important! Here is why:

- warm up is toning all the muscle systems of the body;

- warm up increases cardiovascular activity and stimulates active blood supply to the muscles;

- warmup prevents injuries;

- it increases in intensity and efficiency of training;

- it increases the responsiveness of the nervous system;

- it accelerates metabolic processes;

- it helps to concentrate and creates a proper attitude for training;

- good warm up helps to focus on training, to put off thoughts about the other aside;

- it improves overall and muscle temperature which improves blood circulation in the involved muscles;

- increasing overall and muscle temperatures leads to improved energy production (more strength in training, more spent calories);

- training without a warmup is potential stress for the heart and danger for tendons, ligaments, muscles;

- a heated body is able to show better results than not preheated. Thus it promotes an increase in endurance and strength.

- How long should the warm-up last? 5-10 minutes.Why do you need a stretching after the training session?

After any physical activity, it is important to stop gradually. A sudden stop can cause dizziness, nausea, and fainting. Types of post workout slow down: slow pace walk, jogging, swimming, stretching.

Cardio

Cardio is any kind of physical activity with a high intensity and high heartbeat rate.

What cardio does?

- Improves the functioning of the cardiovascular system;
- Strengthens the heart muscle;
- Improves health;
- Speeds up metabolism;
- Helps to recover more quickly;
- Burns calories and fat.

Why do I run every day for 15-20 minutes, but I do not see any results? The fact is that if the run was short, then the body does not have enough time to "reach" that fat, so it uses energy reserves obtained from food. This explains why cardio should be continuous.

What cardio type is the most effective? You can do rope jumping, swimming, riding a bicycle, but effectiveness is not about the type of the cardio training. It is about intensity and duration.

How to define it whether it is enough intense and enough long? If you just walk on a treadmill for 60 minutes (cardio with low intensity) there will be no real effectiveness! On the contrary, killing yourself so that the heart jumps out of the chest, leads to overwork of the heart muscle. Over time, heart disease can happen. So how do you find the right intensity? For effective cardio (with no harm to your health), you should control your heartbeat rate and keep it within special limits. You can use heart rate monitor or calculate manually.

Cardio Heart Rate (HR) formula:

220 - your age = maximum HR

Your cardio training HR should be within 70 - 90 % of the maximum heart rate.

Before cardio meal goes under same rules as other pre-workout meals we discussed earlier in the chapter "Before and after workout meal".

How to target a problem zone

This is going to be probably the shortest chapter. But I really wanted to include this topic, because a lot of people train to target that one zone that makes them nervous. This can be anything - belly, hips, arms, neck. Does not matter what is your target zone, the truth is that there is NO WAY to change that zone specifically. Many times they advertise that they will tell you how to this, but it is all marketing, nothing to do with real life. In real life, you have to work on your whole body, from head to toes, and your body will change gradually in all zones.

Personal training program

This section is devoted to exercises and training, but first I want to talk with you about some more important things. It is possible that after reading this book you will end up with a problem of information overload about nutrition and fitness. I know that many beginners face this problem. I know that first steps are not that simple. Therefore, you will need to become your personal trainer and contribute to structuring your own life, to build a clear plan of action. Such a plan will help you achieve your goals faster, and your path towards them will be comfortable. Here is another to do list:

Set yourself a goal. It's clear that your goal is a beautiful healthy body, and well-being. But it will be much better if you set intermediate goals and clearly define them. And your goals should have clear boundaries, they should be achievable (for example, if you decided to get rid of cellulite in two weeks, then this is an unattainable goal and it is not good), and it is also necessary to put a clear time frame;

Find what motivates you. For someone, the motivation is a smaller size dress, someone is motivated by photos or video of a famous person, and someone wants to look good on the beach next summer;

Draw up a training plan ahead. You must have a schedule in advance that fits your current pace of life. This will help you to not miss any training;

Plan your training in advance. Since you are your own personal trainer now, you need to come to the gym with a ready training plan, otherwise, your training will not be intense and half the time you will spend thinking about what exercise to do next;

Make changes from time to time. If you do the same exercises all the time, your body learns to adjust to them and the progress of the transformation will stop;

Watch your results. First of all, this is an excellent motivation, when you take a photo before and after and see a difference between them. I'm sure that it creates more desire to eat right and do sports;

Continue to study and find new information. In the literature and Internet sources, there are always more and more new ideas about how to achieve better results. Be aware of them and make changes to your training plan;

Do not forget about proper nutrition. I have already paid enough attention to this topic, but I decided to put this item on the list as it is really very important. All the efforts in the gym will be in vain if you will eat unhealthy food;

Give your body time to recover. Recovery is an important part of the transformation process. Do not forget about the balance between the grand fitness efforts and rational rest. Sometimes it is worth doing stretching, yoga, pilates for good health and further progress;

Only regular efforts will give results. If one week you kill yourself in the gym and eat right, and the next two weeks you go back to your former way of life, then do not expect the result to come. Changes in your body will only happen when from day to day, from month to month, a healthy lifestyle will be a part of you.

Now let's go back to your actual personal training program. It will be good for you, no matter what is your fitness level. This works very simply, but it is uniquely effective. I have been using this method with my clients for several years now and receive wonderful reviews and results. The most important thing is to train regularly. Do not start if you are not ready to train several times a week for at least few months or even years. In fact, proper nutrition is more than enough to feel good and to get attractive, beautiful body. However, if you want to look athletic, increase endurance, strength and temper your cardiovascular system, then read on and apply it as soon as possible.

What I will give you in this section is 50 best exercises for all muscle groups. I suggest to you the method of building bricks. This means that following 50 exercise are those bricks and you take them to build your own workout. Do you remember how you did that in your childhood? You should take 1-2 exercises from each section and build that workout plan. Each time, try to use different exercises in your workouts and do not stuck on the same ones. I've told you before that your body tends to adapt, and this means that if you perform even the best exercise in the world day after day, then one day it will not be effective because your body can now cope with it very easily.

All the exercises are divided into five groups: lower body, upper body, core, cardio, and stretching.

It is very important to remember that before each workout, you need to perform a warm-up. Here is a warm-up that I suggest you do before each workout.

- Neck rotations for 15 seconds
- Shoulder rolls for 30 seconds
- Wide arm circles 30 seconds
- Hip rotations 10 repetitions for each side
- High knees for 30 seconds
- Air squats for 30 seconds
- Lunges 10 repetitions for each side
- Plank 30 seconds

In this training program, all exercises can be performed at home. You will not need any special equipment. If you have a gym membership - it's great and you can do the same exercises in the gym. You can also add group classes to your training plan. For example, Zumba, pilates, yoga, belly dance, stretching. If you feel that you have a lot of strength and energy and want some more activities, then, of course, you can choose other group classes with the use of additional equipment. But keep in mind that overtraining is not good for you.

If at some point your personal training program seems too easy for you, and you do not see any progress, then I recommend starting using additional weights. But you remember I said that training can be done at home without equipment, right? Yes, this is right, at home you can find different things that you can use in your workouts, such as water bottles or heavy books. However, if at some point, even with additional weights your training will not be challenging for you, then this is a sure sign that you need to perform more sets and repetitions. Well, how do you know how many sets and repetitions to add? The answer is very simple: add 10% of the exercise volume of the previous workout. For example, if at the last training you performed 100 squats and you decided to increase the load, then now perform 110 squats. This method will help you smoothly but effectively increase the load when necessary. It is better to add 10 repetitions in each workout than dramatically increase from 100 to 200, and give your body great stress. From such stress, you can get high body temperature, and even get sick.

With each exercise, I give recommended number of repetitions. You can perform all repetitions in one set, or separate to a couple of sets if necessary. You determine the number of sets yourself.

Section 1. LOWER BODY:

1) Step up. In this exercise, you're going to step up on the platform. I'm sure you have a lot of things you can step up on at home. This can be anything from stairs to your sofa. First, you should start from something lower and then move to something higher. Make sure your platform is stable so you stay safe during this exercise. Starting position is face forward to the platform. Step up on it with one leg, go all the way up and then come back. You can help yourself with hands a little bit, but try to focus on your glutes and legs.

Recommended total number of repetitions: 100 each leg

2) Front knee and side leg raise. This exercise will improve your balance and work on the shape of your legs. You might need to stand near the wall to help yourself to find a balance at first, but after a couple of training sessions, you will be able to do this without any help. You should start from moving your knee forward and up, then return it to the starting position, straight your leg and move it up to the side. Ideally, you should not put your foot down to the floor during all exercise. But don't worry if you find it difficult at first.

Recommended total number of repetitions: 60 each leg

3)　　Chair squat and toes rise. I prefer not to include any regular squats into home workout plan because a lot of people are not able to perform them correctly. And incorrect squats will give not any results. So now you know why I choose chair squat. Please choose a chair for this exercise, it should be average height. Starting position in front of the chair. Now start to move down just like you would do this if you wanted to sit on the chair, then reach a chair and go up. After squats, you should continue your movement and go all the way up and do toes rises.

Recommended total number of repetitions: 100

4) Lunges and a front kick. This exercise combines two amazing movements, which will help you to get amazing results. I've been using this exercise many times and to tell you the truth, it is perfect for shredding. We start this move from doing backward lunges, your back leg should go to the comfortable distance so your front knee is just right above your front foot. Then go back to the starting position and keep moving with your opposite leg making a front kick. Please don't try to do a really high kick, it should be done at the comfortable height. This exercise is not about making it high because it is not about stretching. So better concentrate on the pace and work of your muscles.

Recommended total number of repetitions: 80 each leg

5) Glute bridge. Lift your hips off the ground until the moment when your knees, hips, and shoulders are on the same straight line. Squeeze your glutes and keep toned at the top point. I am offering you to do a special bridge. It is special because you have to stop at the top position for three seconds. This will make deep tissues to work. You should go nice and slow, take your time to enjoy the work of muscles. This will help you to concentrate on the work of the muscles better, and feel how they work. I promise you that you will get better results if you visualize and think of your muscles working during each exercise.

Recommended total number of repetitions: 100

6) Side rolling lunges. Starting position: legs are standing wider than shoulders' width. Squat and "roll" to the side lunge. Then roll to another side without standing up. No need to squat deeply, stay at an average level. Knee and toe should look straight. Your knee should not go beyond the foot. Keep your back even and look straight. Roll to the right + roll to the left is 1 repetition.

Recommended total number of repetitions: 80

7) Cross lunges. Starting position legs apart, under shoulders. Cross-step back with one foot.

Front knee on top of the front foot. Keep your back straight, face forward. Return to the starting position. Make a cross-lunge with another leg.

Recommended total number of repetitions: 80 each side

8) Front lunges. This exercise is a lunges "walk". Start moving forward with front lunges all the way through your room and then walk back. Face straight.

Recommended total number of repetitions: 100

9) Side kick. Kick as if you wanted to reach something with your foot. Move at a moderate pace. Help yourself with hands for balance. Your leg should go as high as your stretch allows.

Recommended total number of repetitions: 80 each side

10) Front kick. Perform the same exercise but front direction. Start the movement with your knee and then straight your leg in the top position.

Recommended number of repetitions: 80 each side

Section 2. UPPER BODY:

Usually, women are willing to workout only legs, abs and glutes, and men oppositely like to workout their upper body. But I am sure you know that both genders should develop body proportionally. As I said before, there is no way of getting results in your target area without working out the whole body. So enjoy following upper body exercises.

11) Diagonal wood chop. Starting position: legs are standing as wide as your shoulders' width. Take something in hands. Rise a subject high to one side and then move it down to the opposite with lunge. Your back should be straight at all times and arms should be straight as well.

Recommended total number of repetitions: 50 each side

12) Superman. Starting position laying on the floor face down. Simultaneously raise legs and arms as high as you can, try to hold for 1 second and go back down. If you are not ready to raise both hands and legs, then start from raising arms without legs. You may fix your legs with a sofa, so they stay down at all times.

Recommended total number of repetitions: 20-30

13) Bird. Starting position - on all fours. Simultaneously raise the arm and the opposite leg, so they create one straight line. Hold your arm and

leg at the top for 2-3 seconds and return to the starting position. Do not hold your breath, breathe evenly. Perform at a slow pace. Right hand + left hand = 1 repetition.

Recommended total number of repetitions: 50

14) Biceps curl. Raise dumbbells to the shoulders, once you reach, slowly lower them to a starting position. You should keep elbows stationary burnt all exercise. Do not lift them. Make sure you squeeze bicep on the top position. Fully extend arms at a low position.

Recommended number of repetitions: 80

15) Triceps extension. Hold the dumbbell with both hands behind your head, elbows straight up. Raise dumbbell up and slowly lower it back. Your elbows should remain at the same place during all movement.

Recommended total number of repetitions: 50

Section 3. CORE:

16) Plank. You can do straight hands plank or elbows plank. Both are fine. Keep your body in one straight line. Breathe evenly.

Perform total 120 seconds.

17) Plank steps in. Stand in regular plank, hands are straight. Now start making short steps towards your hands and then go back to the starting position.

Recommended number of repetitions: 50

Section 4. CARDIO:

18) Jumping jacks. Stand with your feet together and your hands down. In one motion jump your feet out to the side and raise your arms above your head. Immediately reverse that motion by jumping back to the starting position.

Recommended number of repetitions: 150

Now I offer you 2 types of Burpees. Sorry, but every workout plan should have this amazing exercise.

19) Burpee #1. Bend over or squat down and place your hands on the floor in front of you, just outside of your feet. Then jump both feet back so that you're now in plank position.3. Drop your body to the floor and push up to return to plank position (this can be a strict push-up or just push yourself up from the ground as you would if you weren't working out). Jump the feet back in toward the hands. Perform one jumping jack and start over again.

Recommended number of repetitions: 30

20) Burpee #2. Repeat everything as in the first variation until you return to a plank position. Now do side kicks with each leg at a time and jump back in toward the hands. Then stand up, and explosively jump into the air, reaching your arms straight overhead.

Recommended number of repetitions: 30

21) Squat and kick. Squat as low as you can and do a side kick. Then squat again and do opposite sidekick.

Recommended number of repetitions: 50 each side

22) Rope jumping. Jump for 30 seconds and then 30 seconds rest.

Recommended total number of rounds: 10

Section 5. STRETCHING:

23) Standing side stretch, butterfly stretch, seated trunk twist

24) Foldover stretch, swan stretch, Standing triceps stretch

25) Seated forward bend, chest stretch, sky reach

Recovery

Recovery

Do you know that pain in the muscles after training, the next day or even a few days after training? Someone worried when imagines how to get out of bed and go to work when everything hurts, and another person thinks that if there is no muscle soreness, then the training was not productive. Now we will figure out what muscle soreness is and discuss the process of recovery. I will talk about methods that will help to recover faster and make this process less painful.

You will be surprised but until now there is no unambiguous opinion about what is the main cause of the muscle soreness. The first theory says that the main reason is a lactic acid which accumulates in muscle tissues during physical work. However, this theory was refused and another scientist suggested the theory of numerous injuries, which says that the muscle soreness is the result of the injuries of the muscle tissues after performing physical work (the fibers are getting broken from heavy loads), and this causes pain.

No matter which theory you choose, you can feel that pain. What to do? The simplest thing you can do when you have muscle soreness is to give your body a natural rest. The muscle soreness will go away by itself in three to five days if you give your body time to restore naturally. It's not about lying on the couch all this time, you just need to live a normal life, but avoid heavy physical work. However, if you want to influence the recovery process and speed it up, here are a few methods:

- Massage. You can go to the massage salon, but if you do not have time for this, then self-massage with a warm-up lotion is also a great option. It is necessary to massage those muscles in the direction of the lymph nodes. For example, massage the hands from the fingers to the shoulders, and the legs from the feet to the hip area. The abdominal muscles must be massaged clockwise.

- Warming gel and compress. Such lotions are sold in pharmacies. You can buy them without a prescription. Apply with massage movements.

- Hot bath, shower or sauna. Under the influence of high temperature, blood vessels dilate and lactic acid is eliminated from the body more quickly. So hot bath, shower or sauna help to prevent or get rid of unpleasant feelings in the muscles.

- Warm up exercises in the open air. The inflow of oxygen will provide intensive blood circulation so after a warm-up in the fresh air you will feel much better. Here we are not talking about intensive training, but about leisurely warm-up or stretching.

Motivation

I decided to sit down and highlight a few "do's and don'ts" that will become your helpers on the way to set goals (not only regarding fitness):

Never give up. Think about efforts that you have already been made. Won't you feel sad for those efforts if you stop now?

Do not criticize yourself or others - it does not help anyone (as a rule), but rather depresses.

Do not let to distract you from your goal. In the middle of the path, it may seem that there is something more interesting or more important or easier. Please stop looking around and stop comparing. If you set that goal it means it was not just born in your head, right? It is what you wanted, so go to on until you reach it.

Do not blame others. May be you are right, and someone else is guilty of something, but take everything in your own hands. Do so because you want changes, not them, and you are able to get them.

Write down goals and objectives - structuring and visualization greatly influence success.

Decide what is your purpose. You cannot spread yourself on many things at the same time. So just decide who you are and what you want this life.

Give success to others. "Outgoing" positive energy waves generate "incoming" ones.

Do not be afraid of change. You can trample on one place if it brings you pleasure, but if not - create a new one!

Generate positive vibes. This positively affects your mind and body.

No reason to wait for the "right" moment, my dear! There always will be a reason, an excuse.

Now I have 2 challenges for you that you should implement in your life as soon as you can. I promise they will not only help to lose weight, get sexy butt and waist but also will bring you closer to the state of harmony with yourself.

Challenge # 1:

Stop trying to please everyone, it is impossible! And there is no point to waste your life energy, vibes and most importantly your time for this. Focus on the really close people: husband, parents, children. Let the others please you, and not vice versa.

It is necessary to change. In the worst case scenario, if you do not like the result, then you can always return to where you started.

Stop to live in the past and stop to let it be a part of your mentality. Such behavior won't let you no notice and enjoy present moments.

Don't be scared of difficulties. Difficulties happen with everyone. There are no people who have everything perfect.

Challenge # 2:

Replace word "dream" with "target", "desire" with "task", "aspiration" with "action".

Conclusion

Remember I told you that you need to be your personal trainer? So now is the time to begin. And I propose to begin with the drawing up of a calendar of training. Print regular calendar, or create one yourself in a format convenient for you, fill in with training in advance and be ready to perform them according to the schedule. I do not know at what level of physical fitness you are now, but I want to offer you a list of goals that you can achieve with regular training, after a while. These goals are kind of rewards for the effort. Choose something that you are interested in and go for it: learn your new abilities, run a marathon, stand in the plank for 3 minutes, learn pull-ups, take part in a bike ride, learn to stand on your hands legs up. I know that now it sounds very difficult, and maybe you think I'm crazy, but believe me, one day, you will feel the power in your body and will do it. The main thing is to set a goal and cheerfully go in its' direction.

I really hope you got enough information and motivation from my book. I tried not to overload with information but provide literally all you might need. If you have a question regarding your diet or training please do not hesitate to contact me at zorinanataly@gmail.com; I want you to be in touch with me because it is important to me that you succeed.

The following and the last section is a healthy recipe book. I know beginners have a hard time to diverse diet, and it turns everything to a very boring process. Since I want you to learn to enjoy staying on a healthy track, so I decide to provide you with those healthy meals to show that it is not about broccoli and plain chicken breast.

Healthy recipe book

it down and enjoy!

CPFC stands for Calories/Protein/Fat/Carbohydrates. Sweet recipes are at the end in case you are looking for them.

OATMEAL VEGETABLE PIZZA

Pizza on the oatmeal pancake is my favorite. Besides, it is cooked quickly. It is good for breakfast/lunch. If it is a bran pancake, it is also good for supper.

CPFC of a plain pancake: 265/ 13.3/ 8.1/ 34

INGREDIENTS FOR A PANCAKE:

- 50g oats

- 1 egg

- 1 teaspoon plain yogurt (or sour cream)

- 40 ml. kefir

- 1/4 teaspoon baking powder

- salt

COOKING:

You just blend all ingredients. Then fry it on a well preheated non-stick frying pan without oil on both sides.

FILLING:

- curd cheese

- green salad

- cucumber

- tomato

- some grated hard cheese

Filling is up to you. Improvise! Done! Enjoy your meal!

CHICKEN ROLLS WITH SUN-DRIED TOMATOES, MOZZARELLA AND SPINACH

CPFC in one roll: 267/ 25/ 14/ 10

INGREDIENTS (for 8 pcs.):

- 8 fine cut slices of chicken fillet

- 1/2 glass sun-dried tomatoes

- 1/2 glass grated mozzarella

- 1/2 glass cut spinach

- 1/4 sliced little red onion

- 1/2 glass seasoned bread crumbs

- 1/4 glass grated Parmesan cheese

- juice of 1 lemon

- 1 tbsp. olive oil

- spray with olive oil

COOKING:

Mix bread crumbs and grated Parmesan cheese in a little bowl. Mix olive oil, lemon juice, and pepper in another bowl. Preheat oven to 225 C. Spray a baking dish with olive oil. Put on every slice of chicken fillet 1 tbsp. each sun-dried tomato, grated mozzarella, spinach and 2-3 slices of red onion. Roll it and place seam side down. Souce it in lemon juice with oil, then in bread crumbs and cheese. Put it in the baking dish. Spray it all with olive oil. Roast during 25 min until cooked and golden - brown. Enjoy your meal!

BROCCOLI CAKE WITH CHICKEN BREAST

I'm sure it will not leave untouched even those people who dislike healthy broccoli.

INGREDIENTS:

- 250 g sour cream

- 250 g chicken fillet

- 200 g white mushrooms

- 2 tbsp. sour cream or natural yogurt

- 1 chicken egg

- 1/2 onion

- chicken spice, salt and pepper

- 70 g hard cheese

COOKING:

Cut broccoli and chicken breast into small pieces, season it with salt and pepper. Mix and leave for 10-15 min. Take a baking dish (you can do it in one big baking dish) and put it in layers: broccoli, chicken pieces, fine cut onion, cut white mushrooms.

FOR SAUCE: mix grated hard cheese with sour cream (natural yogurt) and egg; cover your dish with it and bake it in pots in a preheated 180-200°C oven for 35-40 min. It will be very delicious!

AVOCADO SALAD

It seems that salads are never enough. Besides all benefits, they are made practically from whatever you have at the moment. Healthy salad will "beautify" any table. It adds flavor to main dishes and can be a proper and self-contained meal. Here is one of the best salads:

INGREDIENTS:

- lettuce leaves

- avocado

- tomatoes

- eggs

- marinated in herbs and lemon juice mozzarella

- salt / pepper / herbs

COOKING:

Cut all ingredients. And season with pumpkin seeds oil. It tastes good.

PIZZA WITH RUCCOLA AND SALMON IN 5 MINUTES

INGREDIENTS:

- 2 eggs

- 2 oat bran

- 2 tbsp. porridge oat

- 100 ml. kefir

- salt, pepper

FILLING:

- light curd cheese

- ruccola

- slightly salted salmon

- tomato

COOKING:

Blend all ingredients and bake the pizza base on well preheated non-stick frying pan during 2-3 minutes. Spread a cooked base with curd cheese and filling.

IDEAL DUMPLINGS WITH COTTAGE CHEESE

Dumplings are made of whole-wheat flour with sour cream and jam. There are a few ingredients. It is convenient to cook it for later and refrigerate.

CPFC in a total portion: 664/ 55/ 17/ 86

INGREDIENTS

(for 16-18 pieces, diameter of circles – 8 cm):

- 120g whole-wheat flour

- 1 egg

- 5 ml. olive oil

- vanillin

- 180 cottage cheese

- 30-50 ml. milk

COOKING:

Mix flour (100 g) with vanillin; add oil, warm milk, an egg, and mix. Then cover it with a plastic wrap and leave for 20-30 minutes. Use the rest 20 g flour for sheeting dough. From first of "rested" dough a ball, knead out during 5 min and divide into two parts. Roll out one part until the thickness is about 2 mm. Cut circles with the help of glass/pan. Do the same thing with 2nd part, it must be about 16-20 circles. Fill dumplings with cottage cheese passed through a sieve and mixed with artificial sweetener or any other sweetening product (e.g. honey). Take half a teaspoon of filling. A lot of filling can break dumplings. Seal edges of dumplings accurately. Fill the middle of the circle with filling. You can water edges of dumplings slightly for better adhering. It is necessary to fasten dough tight to avoid falling out of filling during boiling. Throw dumplings into boiling water and cook for about 5-7 min after lifting. Then you can grease it with butter. It will make it tastier. Done! Serve with nonfat sour cream and something sweet! Enjoy your meal!

ONE POT CHICKEN ALFREDO PASTA

Do you like such version of pasta?

INGREDIENTS:

- 1 cut in halves horizontally chicken breast

- 1 tbsp. olive oil

- 250 g pasta

- 2 glasses milk

- 1,5 glass chicken soup

- 1 big fine cut garlic clove

- ½ glass of cream

- ¾ glass grated parmesan

COOKING:

Sprinkle a chicken with salt and pepper. Heat oil in a big frying pan on good fire (you can fry on the non-stick frying pan without oil). Fry chicken until done and golden-brown. Get it out, cover it with a foil and leave for 5 min. Cut it. Reduce fire to medium; add milk, chicken soup, and garlic. Wait until boiling, then add pasta and dip it totally into water. Boil for 10 min, stirring regularly. In 10 minutes pasta will be cooked but still hard. Add cream and parmesan. Boil during 1-2 min until a sauce thickens and pasta becomes al dente (soft but hard). If the sauce becomes too thick, add some hot water and mix it well. Season it with salt and pepper. If you wish to serve it with parmesan and parsley. Enjoy your meal!

CHICKEN WITH VEGETABLES FOR LUNCH OR SUPPER

INGREDIENTS (for 4 persons):

FOR MARINADE SAUCE:

- 450 g cut chicken fillet

- 1 tbsp. soya sauce

- 1 tbsp. sesame oil

- 1 tbsp. maize starch

- 1 tbsp. rice vinegar

- 1 cut in cubes zucchini

- 1 cut in cubes paprika

- ¼ glass peanut

- 8 dried chili

- 3 garlic cloves

- 1 cut bouquet bunching onion

- 2 tbsp. ginger

- 1 tbsp. soya sauce

- 1 tbsp. sugar

- 1 teaspoon rice vinegar

- 2 tbsp. water

- 2 tbsp. maize starch

COOKING:

Mix a chicken with all ingredients for marinade sauce in a medium-sized bowl. Leave it, at least, for 10 minutes. Fry the chicken in an oiled pan on medium heat. Take it out. Add sesame oil, zucchini, and paprika in the frying pan and fry it during 3 minutes. Add peanuts and fry it during 3 minutes. Add dried chili, garlic, ginger, bunching onion and fry till vegetables soften. Add the chicken, soy sauce, rice vinegar, sugar, maize starch (mixed with water) and mix it well. Decorate it with bunching onion and serve with rice. Enjoy your meal!

ASIAN CHICKEN CHOPPED SALAD

INGREDIENTS (for 6 portions):

- 2 chicken breast

FOR MARINADE SAUCE:

- 2 tbsp. soya sauce

- 1 teaspoon sesame oil

- ½ teaspoon black powdered pepper

- ½ teaspoon paprika flakes

- 1 sliced garlic clove

- 1 tbsp. cut ginger

FOR DRESSING:

- ¼ glass rice vinegar

- 1 tbsp. sesame oil

- 1 tbsp. soya souse

- 1 tbsp. sugar

- 1 fine cut garlic clove

- 1 teaspoon grated ginger

FOR SALAD:

- cut cos lettuce

- 1 glass purple cabbage

- ½ glass grated carrot

- ¼ glass bunching onion

- ¼ glass coriander

- ¼ glass almond flakes

COOKING:

Mix all ingredients for marinade sauce in a big bowl. Add chicken breast in the bowl, cover and marinade it in the refrigerator for 30 minutes. Fry the chicken and cut it into cubes. Mix all ingredients for dressing in a jar and shake it well. Add all ingredients for salad in a big bowl, add the chicken and dressing. Mix it and enjoy!

VERY TASTY AND HEALTHY CHEESE SCONES – PERFECT VERSION OF SUGARLESS BREAKFAST OR A SNACK

CPFC in 100 g. 258/ 16/ 10/ 28

Total energy: 892 kcal

INGREDIENTS:

- 130 g whole-wheat flour

- 80 g hard cheese 40%

- 100 g cottage cheese 5%

- 80 ml. kefir 1%

- 10 g butter

- pinch of salt

- 1 teaspoon baking powder

- 1/2 teaspoon soda

- yolk for greasing

COOKING:

Mix flour with butter, baking powder, and soda. Add fine grated cheese, a pinch of salt, cottage cheese, and kefir. Mix all ingredients. It must be a soft dough. Roll it out carefully into a scone to a thickness of 1 cm. Cut it into 8 triangles, grease it with yolk and bake it in a preheated 180 C oven for 20 minutes. Cheese scones are delicious not only warm but also cold. Bon appetite!

CHICKEN SALAD WITH HONEY-MUSTARD DRESSING

INGREDIENTS (for 2 portions):

FOR DRESSING:

- 1,5 tbsp. each Dijon mustard, honey, apple vinegar, olive oil

- 1/4 teaspoon salt + black powdered pepper

FOR SALAD:

- 1 chicken breast + ½ tbsp. oil

- cut lettuce

- 10 cut in halves cherry tomatoes

- 6 asparagus

- ½ cut in circles red onion

- ½ cut avocado

- 50 g cut and fried (if you wish) bacon

COOKING:

Put all ingredients for dressing in a jar and shake it well. Cut a chicken breast in half horizontally, season it with salt and pepper. Grease 2 teaspoons dressing. Heat a non-stick frying pan on good fire. Add asparagus and fry during 3 minutes or until cooked. Take out a frying pan and take it away. Add oil into the pan; fry a chicken during 2 min on both sides or until cooked. Put on a plate, cover with a foil and leave it for 5 minutes. Put lettuce in a bowl and mix it with a little bit of dressing. Put cherry tomatoes, asparagus, avocado, red onion and chicken on top. Strew it with bacon (if you like) and pour rest of dressing. Enjoy your meal!

ROASTED CHICKEN IN HONEY-GARLIC SAUCE

INGREDIENTS:

- 450 g cut into strips chicken fillet

- 2 teaspoon soya sauce

- 1 teaspoon fine cut garlic

- 1 teaspoon grated ginger

- 2 big eggs

- 1 glass bread crumbs or milled oat

FOR SAUCE:

- ⅓ glass honey

- 2 tbsp. soya sauce

- 1 tbsp. Sriracha sauce

- 3 fine cut garlic cloves

- 1 tbsp. water

- 1 tbsp. corn starch

FOR SERVING:

- cut onion

- slightly fried sesame seeds

- french bean

COOKING:

Preheat an oven to 200 C. Cover baking sheet with a parchment. Marinade a chicken fillet in the mixture of soya sauce, garlic and ginger for 15 minutes. Dip the chicken fillet in eggs, then in breadcrumbs or ground oat. Spread it on the baking sheet and bake it till brown and crispy crust for 15 minutes. While the chicken is baking, mix honey, soya sauce, Sriracha sauce and garlic in a saucepan until boil. Add (previously mixed) corn starch and water, mix it till jelling. Pour over the chicken with a sauce and mix it accurately. Serve it with bunching onion, fried sesame seeds and green beans. Enjoy!

PASTA WITH VEGETABLES

Very tasty and quick lunch / supper

INGREDIENTS:

- onion

- mushrooms

- 1 pepper

- 1 carrot

FOR SAUCE:

Mix:

- 3 tbsp. soya sauce

- 1 teaspoon sesame oil

- 1 teaspoon sugar

COOKING:

Boil pasta. Fry onion, mushrooms, pepper and carrot on a small amount of oil. Add lettuce and cooked pasta. Mix it. Add a sauce and mix it once more! Serve and enjoy!

FALAFEL

Falafel is a traditional dish of Israeli cuisine. According to the classic recipe it is cooked in oil but I offer to make it in an oven. Falafel is an ideal snack. Besides it is vegetarian.

CPFC in a total portion: 430 kcal 20 /14/ 60.

Chick-peas contain a lot of protein, thus it is very filling.

INGREDIENTS:

- 100 g dried chickpeas

- 1 garlic clove

- 1 small onion (I took dried onion)

- herbs (coriander, parsley, fennel)

- 1 teaspoon cumin

- 10 ml. olive oil

- 1teaspoon salt

COOKING:

Leave chickpeas in water for 8 hours (it is better for the night). Then boil it (40 minutes). Put chickpeas in a bowl, add cumin and salt, and puree it with the help of blender or masher. It must be a thick. If it is too dry – add some water. Cut onion, garlic and herbs into very small pieces separately. Add it to chickpeas, pour in oil, mix it well and put into the refrigerator for 20 minutes. Preheat an oven to 180-200 C. Cover a baking sheet with a parchment. Form small balls and bake for 25-30 minutes. They have to become brown slightly. Done! Enjoy your meal!

CREAMY COCONUT MATCHA OATMEAL

And how about a tasty coconut and oatmeal for breakfast?

INGREDIENTS (for 2 portions):

- 1,5 glass of water

- 1,5 glass of coconut water

- 1 glass oat flakes

- 2 tbsp. coconut flour

- 2 tbsp. maple syrup

- 2 teaspoon matcha powder

- 1/4 glass coconut flakes

COOKING:

Add water, coconut water and oat flakes in a small saucepan. When boiling, reduce fire and continue to cook until the mixture begins to get thick. Cook during 1 min. Add coconut flour, maple syrup and matcha powder. Continue to boil, stirring it slowly permanently until cooked. Add coconut flakes. Dish it out on plates and decorate !

DELICIOUS CHEESE MUFFINS

INGREDIENTS:

- 3 eggs

- 6 tbsp. flour

- 3 tbsp. cottage cheese

- 1/2 glass yoghurt or kefir

- salt

- 1 teaspoon baking powder

- cheese (cut into strips)

- sesame– if you wish

COOKING:

Whisk eggs with cottage cheese and kefir; add flour, baking powder and salt. Mix it. Dough has to be not thick. Cut cheese. Grease a baking dish; pour out half a dough, put cheese pieces accurately on top (leave edges free), pour out the rest dough, strew it with sesame on top. Bake in a preheated 180 C oven for 40-50 min. Cool it down a little.

SPICY BLACK PEPPER SHRIMP BOWL

INGREDIENTS:

- 450 g shelled large shrimps

- 1 tbsp. olive oil

- 1 teaspoon coconut sugar

- 2 fine cut garlic clove

- 1/2 cut small red onion

- 1 glass sweet peas

- 1 cut in cubes carrot

- 1/2 cut red bell pepper

- 1/2 teaspoon sea-salt

FOR SERVING: steamed brown rice and sesame.

FOR SAUCE:

- ½ teaspoon black powdered pepper

- 3 tbsp. soya sauce

- 1 tbsp. rice wine vinegar

- 1 teaspoon soya sauce

- 3 tbsp. water

- 1 tbsp. Corn starch

COOKING:

Mix all ingredients for a sauce in a small bowl. Take it away. Heat olive oil in a frying pan on medium-heat. Add shrimps, coconut sugar, salt and pepper. Fry it until shrimps become pink on both sides. Take out cooked shrimps and put them aside. Add garlic, peas, red onion, red bell pepper and carrot. Fry it, stirring slowly, until it becomes soft. Add sauce and shrimps, fry quickly while everything doesn't mix up well. Serve it with steamed brown rice and sesame seeds! Enjoy your meal!

ONE POT SUMMER VEGGIE PASTA

INGREDIENTS:

- 1 tbsp. olive oil

- 2 fine cut garlic clove

- 1 cut in cubes small onion

- 3 glass of water

- 340 g Rotini

- 1 yellow squash, cut in half and cut into slices

- 450 g cherry tomatoes

- 1 glass beans

- salt and pepper

- 2 glasses tomato sauce/juice

FOR SERVING: grated parmesan and fresh basil

COOKING:

Heat olive oil in a big frying pan; add onion and garlic. Fry until onion becomes soft. Add all ingredients, except tomato sauce/juice. Salt and pepper it. Cover and cook it within 15 minutes. Remove a cover and cook it for 5 more minutes. Add tomato sauce/juice, mix and serve it with Parmesan and basil. Enjoy your meal!

BAKED CRISPY CHICKEN QUESADILLAS

INGREDIENTS:

FOR CHICKEN:

- 400 g chicken fillet

- 1 teaspoon of each: cumin, paprika, and onion powder

- ½ teaspoon pepper

- ½ teaspoon salt

- 1 tbsp. olive oil

FOR FILLING:

- 1,5 tbsp. olive oil

- ½ small onion

- 1 garlic calve

- 1 paprika and 1 green pepper

FOR FLATBREAD:

- 4 flatbreads

- spray with olive oil

- 1 glass grated cheese

COOKING:

Cut a chicken fillet into small pieces. Cover the chicken with spices and pour it with olive oil. Cut pepper and onion into cubes. Cut garlic in small pieces. Fry onion with pepper. Fry chicken fillet and mix it with vegetables. Spread on the flatbread and sprinkle it with grated cheese. Bake it in a preheated 200-220 C oven for 8 minutes. Overturn it and still bake it for 8 - 10 minutes or to a golden-brown and crispy crust. Serve it at once. Enjoy your meal!

RED BEANS, CHICKEN BREAST AND CROUTONS SALAD

Very tasty, healthy and filling salad for good dinner.

CPFC in 100 g 128/13/4/8

INGREDIENTS:

- 230 g boiled chicken breast

- 200 g   red beans

- 150 g   cucumber pickles

- 50 g (2 loafs) whole-wheat bread

- 10 ml. olive oil

Spices: oregano, dried fennel, basil.

FOR DRESSING: 50 g   sour cream 15% (or natural yogurt)

Pomegranate seeds for decoration.

COOKING:

Boil or roast a chicken breast. You can also fry it on a grill. Cut it into small cubes. I used red beans. You have to strain it through a sieve, let flow down liquid and wash it with water. Add it to a chicken fillet. Cut cucumber pickles in small cubes. Add it to the salad. You can use, of course, ready-made bread croutons but I used home-made. Mix olive oil and spices/herbs . Cut bread into cubes and roll in it in this mixture; leave it for 15 minutes, and then fry it in a dry frying pan. Season salad with 1-2 spoons of nonfat sour cream (or natural yogurt). Add bread croutons at the end. Decorate salad with pomegranate seeds, if you wish.

Bon appetite!

CREAMY LEMONY PASTA

INGREDIENTS:

- 1 asparagus bunch

- 2 fine cut shallot

- 2 fine cut garlic calves

- pinch of fresh thyme

- 1,5 tbsp. mascarpone

- ¼ glass parmesan

- 1 tbsp. olive oil

- 1 tbsp. fresh squeezed lemon juice

- salt and pepper

COOKING:

Cut asparagus stalks. Boil it in slightly salted water. At this time fry shallot and garlic on a frying pan. Add a thyme pinch, salt, and pepper. Add pasta to asparagus, mix it well. Add some mascarpone and mix it well. Serve with a slice of lemon and sprinkle with freshly grated parmesan.

CHOPPED CHICKEN WITH CHAMPIGNONS

Still chewing boiled chicken breast, preparing for summer? Would you like some meatballs? They are just ideal for any meal of the day.

CPFC 113/19.7/7.6/1.3

INGREDIENTS:

- 350 g chicken fillet

-100 g champignons

- 2 egg whites

- 30 g oat bran

- herbs

- salt, pepper

COOKING:

Cut a chicken fillet, champignons, and herbs into small pieces. Blend egg whites with a fork, add salt and pepper. Add oat bran and mix all ingredients. Spread it with a spoon and fry in a non-stick frying pan on both sides.

CHICKEN BREAST STUFFED WITH SUN-DRIED TOMATOES, SPINACH AND CHEESE

INGREDIENTS:

- 2 small chicken breasts

- ½ glass cut into strips sun-dried tomatoes

- 4 thick slices mozzarella

- a bunch of spinach leaves

- 2 teaspoons olive oil

FOR ITALIAN SAUCE:

- 1 tbsp. mustard

- 1 tbsp. white wine vinegar or lemon juice

- ½ teaspoon sugar

- 2 teaspoon olive oil

- ½ teaspoon Italian herbs and paprika flakes

- salt and pepper

COOKING:

Mix all ingredients for the Italian sauce. It will be denser than a usual sauce. Do a pocket in a chicken and grease it with a thick layer of the sauce (including inside). Put sun-dried tomatoes, spinach, and cheese inside. Close the pocket with the help of 2 toothpicks. Heat olive oil (it is possible to fry on the non-stick frying pan) in a frying pan on good fire. Fry the chicken on both sides during 1.5 minutes. Roast it for 15 minutes at 180 C. Leave it for 5 minutes, and then serve. Enjoy your meal!

AJARIAN KHACHAPURI

It is very tasty and filling!

INGREDIENTS:

FOR DOUGH:

- 2 eggs

- 400 g cottage cheese 0%,

- 100 g oat flour

- pinch of salt

FOR FILLING:

- 40 g cottage cheese 0%,

- 100 g of cheese

- 4 eggs

- salt

COOKING:

Take eggs; separate whites from yolks and add cottage cheese, flour and a pinch of salt to the whites. Knead dough by hand, divide it into 4 parts and create a small boat from every part. Grease each boat with the remained yolks and bake it at 180 C for 10 minutes. Mix cottage cheese and grated cheese. Get out the half-cooked boats and lay out a filling in the center. Bake it for about 10 more minutes until cheese melted. Get out khachapuri, place a small raw egg into each boat, salt on top and bake it till done: the white has to get thick, and the yolk remains liquid. Serve it warm. It is correct to eat by breaking off edges of the dough and dipping it in the yolk.

ROASTED BRUSSELS SPROUTS SALAD

INGREDIENTS (for 6-8 portions):

FOR BRUSSELS SPROUTS:

- 450 g Brussels sprouts

- salt and pepper

- 1 teaspoon garlic powder

- 1-2 tbsp. olive oil

FOR DRESSING:

- ¼ glass Greek yogurt

- 2 tbsp. Balsamic vinegar

- 2 tbsp. olive oil

- ½ tbsp. mustard

- 1 fine cut garlic calve

- salt and pepper

FOR SALAD:

- 225 g different greens

- ⅓ glass grated carrot

- ⅓ glass cut almond

- ⅓ glass dried cranberry

- ⅓ glass grated Parmesan

COOKING:

Cut off stalks from Brussels sprouts and cut it in quarters. Put Brussels sprouts in a bowl; add garlic powder, olive oil, salt, and pepper. Oil a baking sheet and spread equally on it a cabbage. Bake it for 20-25 minutes at 200 C. Mix Greek yogurt, balsamic vinegar, olive oil, mustard, grated garlic, salt and pepper for dressing. Put mixed greens, grated carrot, cut almond, dried cranberries, grated Parmesan and baked Brussels sprouts in a big bowl. Pour dressing and mix it well. Enjoy!

CHICKEN IN PINEAPPLE ICING

INGREDIENTS:

- pineapple circles

- half onion (better a red onion)

- 2 kg chicken sticks

- 1 teaspoon salt

- 1 teaspoon pepper

- 1 teaspoon powdered garlic

- 1 teaspoon paprika

FOR ICING:

- 2 glass pineapple juice

- 2 teaspoon chili sauce

- salt and pepper

- 2 teaspoon starch

COOKING:

Preheat an oven to 180 C. Clean and dry up the chicken (with a help of a paper towel). Mix 1 tsp. salt, pepper, garlic powder and paprika. Cut an onion and lay it out on a bottom of a baking pan. Cover the chicken with a mixture of pepper, garlic, and salt. Lay out pineapple pieces. Cover it with a foil and bake it for 25-30 min at 180 C. Remove the foil, increase temperature to 230 C for 15 more minutes to golden-brown.

FOR ICING: Bring juice to boiling in a small saucepan. Continue to boil it until the amount of juice decreases twice. Add chili sauce. Take 3 tbsp. juice from a saucepan and mix it with starch. Place it back in the saucepan with juice. Mix it until gets thick. Add salt, pepper and remove it from the fire. Cover the chicken with pineapple icing. Done!

TASTY AND HEALTHY RYE MINI-PIZZA

INGREDIENTS:

- 150 g whole-wheat flour

- 100 g rye flour

- 2 eggs

- 1 tbsp. olive oil

- 50 g boiling water

- 1/2 tsp baking powder

FOR FILLING:

- 50 g champignons

- 100 g tomatoes

- 30 g light cheese

- 10 black olives

FOR SAUCE:

- 50 g natural yogurt

- 50 g tomato paste

- herbs

COOKING:

Mix flour with the baking powder, add eggs, oil, and salt. Then pour it in boiled water. Knead dough by hand. Cut champignons and vegetables. Mix tomato paste with yogurt and add spices for a sauce. Divide dough into 7-8 parts. Make small pizzas on a silicone mat. Grease it with the sauce and spread a filling. Bake it at 200 C for 30 minutes.

THAI SALAD MADE OF ROAST BEEF, TANGERINE, AND AVOCADO

CPFC:126.3/19.7/4.23/4.41

INGREDIENTS:

- 350 g roast beef

- 1 tangerine

- 1 package salad mix with arugula

- 50 g pomegranate seeds

- 30 ml. soya sauce

- 1 /2 lemon

- 1 avocado

- balsamic cream

- salt and fresh ground pepper

COOKING:

Salt and pepper a beef on every side (oil, if you wish), fry it in the heated frying pan for 1-2 minutes on both sides to a golden-brown. Put meat in the roasting tin, bake it at 200 C for 13-15 minutes depending on the thickness of the roast beef and a desirable condition. Then take it out and cover it with a foil. Leave the meat to rest for 7-10 minutes.

Peel an avocado and tangerine and cut it into small slices. Put lettuce leaves, slices of roast beef, an avocado, tangerine, pomegranate seeds on a plate. Pour it with a sauce of lemon juice and soy sauce. Pour it with balsamic cream before serving.

CAJUN-STYLE CHICKEN SALAD

INGREDIENTS (for 4 portions):

FOR SEASONING:

- 2 tsp paprika

- 1 tsp Cayenne pepper

- 1 tsp garlic powder

- 1 tsp oregano

- 1 tsp thyme

- 1 tsp salt

FOR SALAD:

- 2 chicken breast

- 1 tbsp. olive oil

- 1 cut romaine lettuce

- ½ fine cut red onion

- 1 fine cut avocado

- 285 g cut in halves cherry tomatoes

- 225 g black beans

FOR DRESSING:

- ¼ glass Greek yoghurt

- ¼ tsp grated garlic

- 2 tbsp. lime juice

- 1 tbsp. olive oil

- 1,5 tsp. spices(above)

COOKING:

Preheat an oven to 190 C. Mix all ingredients for seasoning in a small bowl. Leave 1.5 tsp of seasonings for dressing. Grease both parts of chicken breasts with seasoning. Fry a chicken on medium-heat for 4 minutes on both sides in the oiled frying pan, or to golden-brown. Bake it for about 15-20 minutes. Cool it down during several minutes. Mix all ingredients for dressing in a small bowl. Cut chicken in pieces. Put salad, red onion, avocado, cherry tomatoes and black beans in a big bowl. Add the chicken, dressing and mix it well. Enjoy your meal!

ONE PAN CHICKEN BRUSCHETTA

INGREDIENTS (for 4 portions):

- 1 tbsp. olive oil

- ¼ tsp sea-salt

- ⅛ tsp black ground pepper

- 4 chicken breasts, without bones and skin

- 2 fine cut garlic calves

- ⅓ glass balsamic vinegar

- 1 glass cut in halves cherry tomatoes

- 170 g fine cut mozzarella

- 10 basil leaves, for serving

COOKING:

Heat olive oil on medium-heat in a big frying pan. Cover chicken breasts with sea salt and black ground pepper. Add the chicken to a frying pan and fry it until well done and cooked for 4-6 minutes on both sides. Add the fine cut garlic and balsamic to a frying pan and fry it until garlic gives flavor for 1-2 minutes. Put fine cut fresh mozzarella on the chicken breast, cover a frying pan and cook it during 1-2 minutes that cheese melted. Scoop balsamic sauce from a frying pan and put on the chicken. Then add tomatoes to a frying pan. Before serving decorate it with basil leaves.

BEEF WITH BROCCOLI

INGREDIENTS (for 4 portions):

- 1 tbsp. olive oil

- 450 g fine cut beef (flank steak)

- 3 fine cut garlic calves

- 1 fine cut shallot

- 4 fine cut bunching onions

- 4 glasses broccoli

- 2 tbsp. corn starch

- ¾ glass of water

- ⅓ glass soya sauce

- 2 tbsp. coconut / brown sugar

- 1 tsp grated fresh ginger

- ⅛ tsp paprika flakes

COOKING:

Heat oil in a frying pan on medium-heat. Add the beef and fry it until done (6-8 minutes). Take it out from a frying pan and take it away. Put garlic, shallot and bunching onions in the same frying pan. Fry it for 1 minute, stirring often. Add some broccoli, mix it, cover and prepare it within 5 minutes. Mix water and corn starch in a small bowl. Mix it to the cream thickness. Mix soya sauce, brown sugar, ginger and red pepper in other bowl. Add mixture to corn starch and mix it well. Uncover a saucepan and add cooked sauce. Cook the sauce for 3-5 minutes until gets thick. Add the beef, mix it well and prepare it for 2-3 more minutes. Serve it with brown rice!

SALAD OF SHRIMPS AND AVOCADO

INGREDIENTS (for 4-6 portions):

- 450 g medium-sized shelled shrimps

- 1 cut romano salad

- 4 cut in cubes tomatoes

- ½ ginned and cut in cubes jalapenos (if you wish)

- ¼ fine cut red onion

- 2 tbsp. fine cut cilantro

- 1 big avocado, cut in cubes

- ½ tsp salt

- 1 rich lime(2 tbsp. juice)

- oil for frying (it is better to fry on anti-adherent frying pan without oil)

Spice mix:

- ½ tsp salt

- ½ tsp black ground pepper

- 1tsp ground thyme

- 1 tsp dried oregano

- ¼ tsp garlic powder

- ½ tsp chili powder

COOKING:

Heat oil in a frying pan on medium-heat (better without oil). Put shrimps with spice mix. Fry it for about 2 minutes. Remove it from fire. Mix salad, shrimps, tomatoes, jalapenos, red onion, cilantro, avocado, salt and lime juice well in a big bowl. Serve it with tortilla or taco. Enjoy!

CREAM OF CHICKEN SOUP

How about such version of lunch?

INGREDIENTS:

- 100 g chicken fillet

- 30 g porridge oat

- 200 g cauliflower

- fresh and dried herbs

- salt / pepper – paprika, Cayenne pepper

- 1-2 croutons

COOKING:

Cook chicken, porridge oat and cauliflower together in a saucepan. Add herbs, spices, salt / pepper to soup. Blend soup until smooth, pour it on plates and decorate it with the broken croutons and spices.

RICE WITH MEAT AND VEGETABLES

INGREDIENTS:

- 450 g cut chicken breasts

- salt and pepper

- 450 g broccoli

- 225 g cut mushrooms

- oil for frying

FOR SAUCE:

- 3 fine cut garlic cloves

- 1 tbsp. grated ginger

- 2 tbsp. sesame oil

- ⅓ glass soya sauce

- 1 tbsp. brown sugar

- 1 glass chicken stock

- ¼ glass flour

COOKING:

Fry a chicken with salt and pepper until done and golden-brown in a big frying pan on medium-heat. Take out cooked chicken from a frying pan and put it aside. Add mushrooms to the same frying pan. Add some broccoli and fry it until done and soften slightly. Take out mushrooms and broccoli from a frying pan. Add 1 tbsp. of oil, garlic and ginger to a frying pan. Then add other ingredients for a sauce and mix it until smooth. Put chicken and vegetables in a frying pan to the sauce and mix it well. Serve with rice or noodles. Enjoy your meal!

MEATBALLS IN CRANBERRY SAUCE

CPFC in 100 g: 189.8/12.84/13.97/2.43

CPFC sauce in 100 g: 58.95/0.62/0.04/14.58

FOR MEATBALLS:

- 300 g minced meat

- 1 big onion

- 1 egg

- 3 tsp oat bran

- milk

- salt, pepper, spices

FOR SAUCE:

- 200 g cranberry

- 2 tbsp. soya sauce

- 1 tbsp. sugar (artificial sweetener, honey)

- cinnamon

- some water (about5 tbsp.)

- juice of 1 orange

COOKING:

Put oat bran in warm milk so that it is like a gruel. Mix all ingredients, form meatballs and fry it in a frying pan without oil to golden-brown. Put it in the clean frying pan. Sauce preparation: mix all ingredients and cook it for about 7-10 minutes till thick. Pour it out on meatballs and steam it under a cover for 5 more minutes. Rice will be a perfect side dish. Bon appetite.

STUFFED PEPPERS

INGREDIENTS (for 6 portions):

- 1 tbsp. olive oil

- 675 g minced beef

- 1 cut in cubes onion

- 2 fine cut garlic calves

- 1 tsp sea salt

- 1/2 tsp black ground pepper

- 1 tsp paprika

- 1 tsp chili powder

- 1/2 tsp dried oregano

- 1,5 glass brown rice

- 3 glass chicken stock

- 200 g cut in cubes tomatoes

- 225 g tomato paste

- 6 medium-sized sweet peppers (red or green)

- 2 tbsp. grated parmesan

- parsley (for serving)

COOKING:

Preheat an oven to 175 C. Pour in brown rice with chicken stock in a deep saucepan and cook it on low heat under the closed cover for about 20 minutes or until cooked. Heat olive oil in a big and deep frying pan on medium-heat. Add minced beef, an onion, garlic, sea salt, black ground pepper, chili powder, dried oregano, paprika and mix it well. Fry it until meat becomes rosy and onion softens (6-8 minutes). Then add tomatoes, tomato paste, cooked brown rice (3 glasses) and mix it well. Wash peppers, cut off tops and take all insides away. Put peppers in a baking dish, fill it with a mixture of rice and minced meat, strew it with grated cheese parmesan on top. Bake it for 45 minutes or till peppers become soft. Bon appetite!

ROLL OF BURRITO BREAD WITH COTTAGE CHEESE AND HARD CHEESE

INGREDIENTS:

- thin burrito bread

- cottage cheese

- grated cheese

- 2 garlic calves

- herbs

COOKING:

Mix cottage cheese, grated hard cheese, fine cut garlic and very small chopped herbs (fennel). Spread burrito with a cheese stuffing carefully and completely. Roll lavash in a thick roll accurately. Press it down by hand. Spread it on a baking sheet and bake it at 190 C, approximately for 10 minutes. Grease roll with a yolk for golden-brown in 5 min until done. Take out cooked roll from the oven, cool it down. Serve it up beautifully!

GRILLED HALLOUMI WITH POMEGRANATE SALAD

INGREDIENTS:

- 2 tbsp. mustard

- 1 tbsp. white wine vinegar

- 2 tbsp. olive oil

- 1 tsp. pomegranate juice/honey

- 250 g halloumi cheese

- 100 g pomegranate seeds

- 100 g arugula

- mint leaves, for serving

COOKING:

Make dressing in a small bowl. Mix mustard with pomegranate juice or honey, vinegar and oil for this purpose. Heat a frying pan on high heat. Cut cheese into 8-10 slices and fry it in a dry frying pan within 1-2 minutes on both sides until it darkens and begins to melt. Spread arugula on a plate and put cheese on top. Pour dressing, and sprinkle pomegranate seeds and mint leaves. It is served at once with a warm pita. Bon appetite!

OMELETTE WITH RICE

INGREDIENTS:

FOR OMELETTE:

- 3 eggs

- 2 tbsp. water

- 1 tbsp. sunflower oil

FOR RICE:

- 120 g boiled rice

- 50 g ground pork

- 1/6 onion

- 1/2 small tomato

- 2 green beans

- 1 grated garlic clove

- 1 tbsp. sunflower oil

- 2 tbsp. tomato paste

- 1 tbsp. oyster sauce

- 2 tsp. fish sauce

- 1/2 tsp. sugar

FOR SERVING:

- chili sauce

- lettuce

- bunching onion

COOKING:

Cut an onion, tomatoes and green beans in cubes. Heat some sunflower oil in a frying pan. Fry a garlic and onion till golden-brown. Then add ground pork, tomatoes, and green beans and fry it until cooked. Add cooked rice, tomato paste, fish sauce, oyster sauce, sugar and fry it for 1 minute.

Switch off fire and take pan away. Mix eggs and water in a bowl. Heat some sunflower oil in a big frying pan. Pour out eggs there. Put rice there when the omelet is cooked. Also wrap an omelet. Serve it with lettuce leaves, green onions and chili sauce. Bon appetite!

TURKEY WITH CHAMPIGNONS IN SAUCE BECHAMEL

Quick, simple and juicy.

INGREDIENTS:

- 400g turkey breast

- 150 g champignons (cut in thin circles)

- 1 egg

- 1 glass of milk

- 150 g mozzarella

- 1tbsp. flour

- 30g butter

- salt, black ground pepper, nutmeg

COOKING:

Put turkey (chicken) breasts in a roasting tin. Salt and pepper it. Put mushrooms on top. Cooking of béchamel sauce: melt butter on low-heat, add a spoon of flour and mix it so there were no curds. Heat milk slightly; pour it out to oil and flour. Mix it well. Salt and pepper it. Add nutmeg. Cook it 2 more minutes (milk shouldn't boil, mix it constantly). Remove it from fire and add an egg. Mix it well. Fill in breasts with mushrooms. Cover it with a foil and roast it at 180C for 30 minutes. Remove foil in 30 minutes and sprinkle it with cheese. Roast it for 15 more minutes. Bon appetite!

BAKED EGG IN AVOCADO

INGREDIENTS:

- 2 avocados

- 4 eggs

- 4 tbsp. grated mozzarella

- 2 slices of fried and cut bacon (if you wish)

- salt, pepper

COOKING:

Heat an oven to 215 C. Cut an avocado in half. With the help of a tablespoon put out pulp (more or less, depending on preferences, the eggs and avocado sizes) from the avocado. Place avocado halves in a baking dish and fill with a mix of 1 egg and avocado in each half of the avocado accurately. Sprinkle cheese on top, put bacon and salt, pepper. Bake it at 215 C within 14-16 minutes until cooked. Serve it with the crushed herbs.

SALMON WITH CITRUS SAUCE AND MINT LEAVES

INGREDIENTS:

- 2 slices of salmon 150 g each

- 3 oranges

- lemon

- 1 tbsp. rice flour or starch

- 1 pinch of curcuma

- salt, black ground pepper

- 1 tbsp. olive oil

- mint for serving

COOKING:

Sprinkle fish with salt and pepper, add some olive oil and marinade it for 20 minutes. Fry it on a frying pan within 10-15 minutes. Squeeze orange and lemon into a small bowl; add turmeric and flour. Mix it well and pour it out in the same frying pan. Stir it slowly until a sauce is thick. Sauce the fish and decorate it with mint leaves.

SALMON WITH BROCCOLI

INGREDIENTS (for 2 portions):

FOR SALMON:

- 1 tbsp. sunflower oil

- ¼ cup maple syrup

- 2 tbsp orange juice

- 2 tbsp. soya sauce

- 1 tsp. ground ginger

- 1 grated garlic clove

- salt and pepper

- 2 salmon fillets

- fresh parsley, for serving

FOR BROCCOLI:

- salt

- 450 g broccoli

- 2 tbsp. butter

- 1 tbsp. soya sauce

- 1 grated garlic clove

- 1 tsp. lemon juice

- 1 tsp. paprika flakes

COOKING:

Fill an average pan with water and cook broccoli there. Add a pinch of salt and boil it. Mix maple syrup, orange juice, soya sauce, garlic, salt and pepper in a bowl. Leave 2 tablespoons of marinade for serving. Place a salmon fillet in a bowl with marinade and dip it well. Fry salmon on a frying pan for 2-3 minutes on both sides using olive oil. Cooked broccoli wash with cold water. Dry broccoli, spread it on a frying pan, add butter, soya sauce, garlic, lemon zest, paprika flakes, mix it well and fry on low-heat for 30-60 seconds stirring it constantly. Spread broccoli and salmon fillet on each plate and pour it with the rest of marinade. Enjoy your meal!

MINI SPINACH ARTICHOKE FRITTATAS

INGREDIENTS:

- 1 tbsp. olive oil

- 400 g dried and cut artichoke

- 3 grated garlic cloves

- 5 cups spinach

- 8 eggs

- 4 cut slices of bacon

- 1/3 cup cottage cheese

- 1/3 cup almond milk

- 1/4 tsp. black ground pepper

- 1/3 cup grated parmesan

COOKING:

Preheat an oven to 175 C. Put oil in a baking dish, heat olive oil on medium-heat and add cut artichokes. Stir it slowly often until it is brown (about 3-4 minutes). Then add garlic and cook it 1 more minute. Add spinach and cook it, keep stirring constantly for about 1-2 minutes. Cool it down. Place eggs in a big bowl. Add the spinach mix, bacon, cottage cheese, milk, black ground pepper and mix it well. Put it in the prepared baking dish. Sprinkle each cake with grated parmesan. Bake it within 25 minutes, till it is golden brown.

CHICKEN IN TOMATO SAUCE

INGREDIENTS (4 portions):

- 4 chicken fillets
- ½ cut paprika
- ½ cut green pepper
- ½ cut yellow pepper
- ½ cut red onion
- ½ lime
- ½ jar tomato sauce
- 75 g grated cheese

FOR SEASONING:

- 1 tsp. paprika
- 1 tsp. cumin
- 1 tsp. garlic powder
- 1 tsp. Cayenne pepper
- 1 tsp. ground cilantro
- ½ tsp. salt
- ½ tsp. black ground pepper

COOKING:

Preheat oven to 180 C. Mix all ingredients for seasoning in a small bowl. Place chicken breasts in a square baking dish and sprinkle with seasoning on top. Pour out tomato sauce on the fillet, spread pepper and onions on top. Squeeze lime juice equally on a chicken, then sprinkle seasoning once again as necessary. Sprinkle cheese on top and bake it within 30-45 minutes or until done. Serve it and enjoy your meal!

CHICKEN PASTA WITH AVOCADO SAUCE

INGREDIENTS (for 6-8 portions):

- 2 cups fresh basil leaves

- 1 big ripe avocado

- 4 garlic cloves

- ¼ glass of walnuts

- 4 tbsp. freshly squeezed lemon juice

- 1 tbsp. water (if you wish – more)

- ½ glass grated parmesan

COOKING:

Blend basil leaves, an avocado, garlic, walnuts and lemon juice in the blender. Add water until the texture of the sauce becomes smooth. Add grated parmesan. Keep sauce in the refrigerator. Spread this sauce over cooked chicken breasts to add new taste.

FRITTATA WITH SWEET POTATOES

INGREDIENTS:

- 3 yolks

- 4 egg whites

- 1 small sweet potatoes cut into cubes

- 2 tsp. olive oil

- 1 small onion cut into cubes

- 2 cups cut kale leaves (or spinach)

- 1 glass of water

- salt and pepper

COOKING:

Mix 3 yolks and 4 egg whites. Preheat an oven to 230 C. Mix sweet potatoes with 1 glass of water in a frying pan. Bring it to boiling condition, reduce fire and cook, stirring it slowly until all water evaporates and sweet potatoes become soft (about 8 minutes). As soon as water evaporates, add olive oil, onion, salt, pepper and mix it. Fry it on medium-heat, stirring it slowly until onion softens. Add cut kale/spinach and fry it, stirring slowly (2-3 minutes). Distribute vegetables evenly on a baking dish, pour out egg mixture on top. Bake it in the preheated oven (5-6 minutes).

CHICKEN AND VEGETABLE TORTILLA

INGREDIENTS:

FOR SEASONING:

- 2 tsp. chili powder

- 1,5 tsp. ground cumin

- 1 tsp paprika

- 1/2 tsp. ground cilantro

- salt and black ground pepper

FOR FILLING:

- 700 g thick strips chicken fillet (2,5 cm each)

- 3 peppers cut into strips (red, green and yellow)

- 1 cut medium-sized onion

- 2 grated garlic cloves

- olive oil

- 2 tbsp. fresh lemon juice

- 3 tbsp. cut cilantro

FOR SERVING:

- 8 tacos / tortillas

- sour cream

- herbs

- avocado, tomatoes, cheese

COOKING:

Heat an oven to 200 C. Sprinkle some oil on a baking sheet.

For seasoning, mix chili powder, cumin, paprika, cilantro, salt and black ground pepper in a small bowl. Spread pepper and onions on a baking sheet. Put strips of the chicken fillet on top, then add garlic and spread seasoning evenly. Sprinkle with olive oil as well. Mix everything well and put it evenly on a baking sheet. Bake in preheated oven for 20-25 minutes until vegetables become soft and the fillet is cooked. Try not to over dry chicken. Get baking dish from the oven, pour it with lime juice evenly, sprinkle cilantro, salt and mix it. Fill tortilla with stuffing and serve it! Bon appetite.

TUNA AND GRAPEFRUIT SALAD

It is ideal for tasty and healthy lunch or dinner.

INGREDIENTS (for 1 person):

- 150 g arugula

- 100 g tuna

- half a grapefruit

- 2 tbsp. sesame

- olive oil and wine vinegar for dressing

COOKING:

Cut tuna, roll in sesame, salt and fry slightly in a dry frying pan. Peel grapefruit and divide to pieces. Mix fish and grapefruit with arugula, add oil and vinegar.

ROAST BEEF SALAD

INGREDIENTS (for 2 portions):

- 100 g mix salad

- 100 g. oyster mushrooms

- 100-200 g roasted beef

- 3-4 sun-dried tomatoes

- 1 tbsp. Sesame seeds

- olive oil

- salt

- pepper

COOKING:

Fry/ bake oyster mushrooms. Cut a roast beef into very thin pieces. Cut dried tomatoes in small pieces. Fry sesame on high-heat for 1 minute. Spread lettuce leaves, oyster mushrooms, dried tomatoes, and roasted beef on plates. Season it with oil, salt, pepper and sprinkle sesame.

BROCCOLI AND CAULIFLOWER PASTA CASSEROLE

INGREDIENTS:

- 500g tagliatelle (pasta)

- 2-3 carrots

- 1 big onion

- 200 g cauliflower

- 200 g broccoli

- 50 g semolina

- 2 big eggs

- salt, pepper

- cheese

COOKING:

Boil pasta until cooked. Cut onion and grate the carrot. Fry onion with carrots during 3 minutes until soft, then mix it with pasta. Cut florets of cauliflower, boil it until soft, do the same with broccoli. Mix pasta, onion, carrot, broccoli, cauliflower, semolina, and eggs. Add salt and pepper. Sprinkle it with grated cheese and bake it in the oven at 180 C for 30-35 minutes. Cheese can be added at the end. Bon appetite!

MUSHROOM PIE

It is a super chicken pie with mushrooms.

INGREDIENTS:

PIE BASE:

- 1 egg

- 2 egg white

- 100 ml. kefir

- 1 glass(240 ml.) buckwheat flour (or another kind)

- 1/2 tsp baking powder

- salt

FILLING:

- boiled chicken breast

- mushrooms

- raw egg white

- nonfat cheese

- herbs

COOKING:

Mix eggs with the mixer, add salt. Add kefir, shake it all. Mix flour, salt, and baking powder and then pour it gradually in egg mix. Make dough. Leave it in the refrigerator for 20 minutes. Stew mushrooms on a frying pan, then cool it. Add egg white and grated cheese. Distribute dough on the baking sheet. Lay out a breast, mushrooms and then herbs. Bake it at 180 C for 20 minutes.

BAKED TILAPIA FILLET IN AVOCADO SAUCE

INGREDIENTS:

FOR TILAPIA:

- 450 g tilapia fillet

- 1 tbsp. ground chili pepper

- 1 tsp cumin

- 1 tsp Cayenne pepper

- ½ tsp salt

- ½ tsp black ground pepper

- 1 tbsp. lime juice

- 1 tbsp. olive oil

FOR SAUCE:

- 1 avocado

- ½ glass cut cilantro

- ½ tsp salt

- ½ tsp. black ground pepper

- 1 tbsp. lime juice

- ¼ cup Greek yogurt

COOKING:

Preheat an oven to 200 C. Mix ground chili pepper, cumin, Cayenne pepper, salt, black ground pepper with lime juice and olive oil in a small bowl. With the help of a brush grease properly each part of the tilapia fillet with marinade. Bake fish for 12 minutes (or until done) in the preheated oven. While the fish is baked, prepare a sauce. Mix avocado, cilantro, salt, pepper, lemon juice and the Greek yogurt using a blender. Mix it until mixture becomes smooth. Place sauce on top of the tilapia fillet and decorate it with fresh cut cilantro. Enjoy your meal!

SHAKSHUKA

INGREDIENTS (for 2 portions):

- 4 eggs

- 2 tbsp. olive oil

- 1 medium-sized onion

- 1 sweet pepper

- 2 garlic cloves

- 600 g tomatoes in own juice or fresh tomatoes

- fresh parsley

- dried paprika

- red hot pepper

- oregano

- salt

COOKING:

Fry onion and garlic in a pan till it is golden-brown. Add chopped sweet pepper later. Cook for 2-3 more minutes. Cut large tomatoes, spread it in a frying pan together with the chopped herbs, seasonings and keep it on medium-heat for 5-7 minutes. I used 300 g canned tomatoes and 2 small fresh tomatoes. Add salt and pepper, then dried oregano. After that, reduce fire, make wholes in the vegetable mash and add 4 eggs there, try not to damage yolks. Cook it on low heat until whites will be cooked and yolks remain liquid. Sprinkle fresh parsley on top.

AVOCADO SALMON SALAD

CPFC in 100 g. 186/11.7/13.9/2.8

INGREDIENTS:

- Lettuce leaves

- 70 g slightly salted salmon

- half avocado (70 g)

- 1 egg

COOKING:

Cut and mix all ingredients. Use balsamic cream sauce as dressing.

BROWN RICE WITH TURKEY AND BROCCOLI

INGREDIENTS:

- 100 g brown rice

- 250 g turkey fillet

- 200 g broccoli

- leek

- 3 tbsp. soya sauce

- parsley or cilantro

- coriander

- salt

COOKING:

Keep brown rice in water for several hours. Then boil it until cooked and keep it under the lid for another 30 minutes. Fry turkey fillet together with onions until golden-brown, then add broccoli, pepper, coriander and fry it on medium-heat, stirring it constantly for 5-7 minutes. Then add rice, soya sauce, and parsley. Cook all together for about 1-2 minutes.

ORANGE CHICKEN

Do you like a sweet-salty combination? I am just in love with this recipe.

INGREDIENTS:

- 550g chicken

- 2 small oranges

- 1 lemon

- 2 small onion

- 1 tsp. olive oil

- thyme

- artificial sweetener

- salt, pepper

COOKING:

Mix juice of one orange, lemon juice, oil, sweetener, salt and pepper in a cup. Cut an onion, divide orange to pieces and put them together with chicken in a bowl. Pour it with just made dressing on top, sprinkle some thyme and leave it for several hours. Then spread all on a baking sheet, wrap it up with a foil and bake it for 30 minutes at 180 C. Then remove foil and bake it for another 10-15 minutes.

SALAD WITH BAKED VEGETABLES AND AVOCADO SAUCE

INGREDIENTS (for 4 portions):

- 1 paprika;

- 500 g. squash or sweet potatoes

- 500 g Brussels cabbage sprouts

- 2 tsp. dried oregano

- 1 tsp salt

- 1 tsp black ground pepper

- 3 tbsp. olive oil

- 100 g. different herbs

DRESSING WITH AVOCADO:

- 1 avocado;

- 1 small garlic clove;

- juice of 1 lime;

- 1/4 cup olive oil;

- 1/2 tsp salt;

- 1/4 tsp. black ground pepper.

COOKING:

Preheat an oven to 200 C. Mix squash or sweet potatoes, red pepper, Brussels sprouts, dried oregano, salt, black ground pepper and olive oil in a big bowl. Lay out vegetables on a baking sheet in one layer and bake it for about 40 minutes. Mix avocado, garlic, lemon juice, olive oil, salt and black ground pepper in the blender until smooth. Spread dressing over squash and serve it nicely. Enjoy your meal!

SHRIMPS AND AVOCADO SALAD

INGREDIENTS:

- 500 g shrimps

- 1 avocado

- 2 tomatoes

- 1 sweet pepper

- green salad

- olive oil

- 4 tbsp. nuts

- balsamic vinegar

- salt

- black ground pepper

- 10 g butter

- ½ sweet red onion

- ¼ lemon

COOKING:

Peel shrimps and dry them with a paper towel. Fry shrimps on butter. To make them slightly roasted – it is enough to cook them for approximately 3- 5 minutes on high-heat. Take shrimps away and cool them down a little. Spray lemon juice on shrimps. Wash green salad. Cut tomatoes in small cubes. Cut paprika (red, orange or yellow). Divide avocado into 2 parts, then cut. Sprinkle lemon juice on it. It is better to use red sweet onion. Cut onion into rings. Mix all ingredients for dressing in a big bowl and season a salad. As for dressing, it is good to use olive oil, balsamic vinegar, salt and spices. It is possible to season it in a big bowl or to pour every portion separately, sprinkling nuts on top. Bon appetite!

CHERRY CHICKEN

MARINADE:

- 100g fresh cherries

- 500g chicken fillet

- 100 ml. soya sauce

- juice of 1/2 lemon

- 2 garlic cloves (cut into large pieces)

- 4 tbsp. honey

COOKING:

Mix all ingredients and add the cut in pieces chicken fillet. Marinade it for 1 hour. Heat frying pan well, dry chicken pieces with a paper towel, fry it quickly and take it out on a plate. Add marinade to the same frying pan and evaporate water until it is thick. Add chicken, mix and fry for couple more minutes. Add cherries before serving.

AVOCADO SALAD

INGREDIENTS:

- arugula

- tomato

- 1/2 avocado

- 3 slices of fresh mozzarella

- basil leaves

- 1 tbsp. olive oil

- 1,5 tsp. Balsamic vinegar

- 1 tsp. honey

- salt and pepper

COOKING:

Mix mozzarella, tomatoes, arugula and avocado in a bowl. Add basil leaves on top. Mix olive oil with balsamic vinegar in a small bowl, add sugar or honey, salt, and pepper. Season your salad with this sauce. Enjoy!

CELERY CABBAGE SALAD WITH CORN, TURKEY, AND BALSAMIC DRESSING

INGREDIENTS:

- Greek yogurt

- celery

- tomato

- corn

- cucumber

- grilled turkey fillet

- salt and herbs

COOKING:

Cut all ingredients and season it with Greek yogurt and balsamic vinegar. Sprinkle it with sesame seeds.

CHICKEN BREAST AND AVOCADO ROLL

It is very tasty and filling!

INGREDIENTS:

- boiled chicken breast

- burrito bread

- avocado

- sour cream 15-20% fat

- cheese

- garlic

- egg

- salt, pepper

COOKING:

Grate avocado, cut cooked chicken fillet, add 3 tsp of sour cream, garlic and mix it all well. Lay out this mix on burrito bread and roll it. Beat the egg in a bowl. Roll your burrito rolls in the egg, then bake it for 5-7 minutes in the oven. Bon appetite!

ROASTED CHICKEN BREAST WITH ASPARAGUS

INGREDIENTS:

- 2 chicken fillets

- 1 asparagus bunch

- green onion

- 4 garlic cloves

- 1 tbsp. soya sauce

- 1 tbsp. honey

- 1 tbsp. olive oil

- sesame seeds

- sesame oil

COOKING:

Cut chicken breast into small pieces. Mix honey and soy sauce in a bowl, then place chicken in it. Mix it thoroughly and put into the refrigerator. Warm up oil in a big frying pan. Cut and fry asparagus within 5 minutes. Take out asparagus from a frying pan. Take out the chicken from marinade; fry it for about 5 minutes on the same pan. Add garlic, green onion and left marinade. Cook it for another 3 minutes. Remove it from fire, add sesame oil and mix it. Serve it with rice. Bon appetite!

AVOCADO AND CHAMPIGNONS SALAD

Delicious and healthy salad.

INGREDIENTS:

- lettuce / arugula

- soft avocado

- cherry tomatoes

- 150 g champignons

- pine nuts

- juice of 1/4 lemon

COOKING:

Cut champignons and fry them slightly on a drop of oil or without it. Sprinkle lemon juice when cooked. Cut tomatoes in half. Cut avocado into small cubes and sprinkle lemon juice on it. Mix champignons with salad leaves/arugula, cherry tomatoes, and avocado. Add salt and pepper, then sprinkle pine nuts on top before serving.

CREAMY PASTA WITH TURKEY

INGREDIENTS (for 1 portion):

- 50 g spaghetti,

- 150 g turkey fillet or chicken

- 100 ml. Cream (10% fat)

- 1 carrot

- 1 onion

- spices

COOKING:

Marinade meat in spices for 1 hour. Grate carrot and cut onion. Stew it on a frying pan for 7-8 min. until all water is evaporated. Add a turkey to vegetables and fry it for 7-8 more min. Boil spaghetti at the same time. Pour out cream and spaghetti in a frying pan, when meat is cooked well inside. Add spices if you like. Cook it all together for another 5-7 mins.

AVOCADO CARBONARA

INGREDIENTS (for 2-3 portions):

- 1 avocado

- 1 egg yolk

- ½ glass thick cream

- 1 garlic clove

- ½ lemon juice

- ½ cup grated parmesan

- 100g chicken fillet

- 250 g spaghetti

- 1 tbsp. olive oil

COOKING:

Blend avocado, egg yolk, garlic and lemon juice using the blender. Then add rich cream and mix it until smooth. Boil chicken fillet. Cook spaghetti at the same time. Add olive oil in cooked spaghetti. Add sauce, chicken, parmesan, salt and pepper, mix it well. Enjoy! Bon appetite!

FILLET ROLLS WITH CHEESE AND ROSEMARY IN MILK SAUCE

INGREDIENTS:

- 3 (700 g) turkey (chicken) fillet

- 2-3 garlic cloves

- 100 g cheese (ideally low fat)

- 3-6 thin slices of prosciutto

- 1-2 tsp rosemary

- 500 ml. skimmed milk

- 1 tbsp. corn starch

- salt

- fresh-ground pepper

- 1/2 tsp nutmeg

- 2-3 tsp paprika

COOKING:

Heat oven to 200 C. Beat off a fillet on both sides, add salt and pepper. Then squeeze out garlic on top and distribute it evenly on the meat. Sprinkle rosemary and paprika. Dice cheese and lay it out on meat. Make rolls, wrap up each roll with prosciutto slices and pin a toothpick through. Lay rolls out on a baking sheet. Mix milk with corn starch, salt, pepper, and nutmeg in a pan, warm it up and stew. Cover rolls with this sauce and bake it for about 25-30 minutes. Sprinkle rosemary before serving. Bon appetite!

BRIGHT AND UNUSUAL PERSIMMON ARUGULA SALAD

INGREDIENTS:

- 2 persimmons

- 0,5 glass almond flakes

- arugula

- salt

FOR SAUCE:

- 2 tbsp. olive oil

- 1 tbsp. Balsamic vinegar

- 1 tsp. liquid honey

- salt

- fresh-ground black pepper

COOKING:

Cut persimmons. Dry almonds on a dry frying pan. Wash arugula and dry it on a paper towel. Combine all ingredients for a sauce in a bowl and shake up it slightly with a wire whisk. Lay out arugula in a salad bowl, add persimmons, pour it with sauce, mix salad and sprinkle with almonds. Bon appetite!

CABBAGE STEW WITH CHAMPIGNONS

INGREDIENTS:

- cabbage

- champignons

- tomato paste

- salt, black ground pepper, bay leaves

COOKING:

Chop cabbage, cut mushrooms, put everything in a pan and pour some water on it. Cover and stew it for about 10 min., periodically stirring slowly. Add half a glass of water to tomato paste, pour in cabbage with mushrooms, add salt and pepper. Add a couple of bay leaves and stew it slowly 10 more min. under a cover on low-heat. The main thing is not to overcook.

CHICKEN WITH VEGETABLES AND PESTO

INGREDIENTS (for 4 portions):

- 2 tbsp. olive oil (or you can fry without oil)

- 4 chicken leg quarters, without bones and skin (replace with fillets if you want)

- salt and pepper

- 450 g. Green beans

- 2 cups cut in halves cherry tomatoes

- ½ cup of pesto sauce

COOKING:

Heat olive oil in a big frying pan and add chicken thighs (or a fillet). Season it with salt and pepper. When the chicken is fried thoroughly, put it on a plate, cut it in strips. Add green beans to a frying pan and cook it until golden-brown. Add chicken to a frying pan, then add tomatoes and pesto sauce. Mix it and cook 2-3 more minutes. Enjoy your meal!

CHICKEN WITH VEGETABLES

INGREDIENTS:

- 400 g chicken fillet

- 200 g broccoli

- 200 g cauliflower

- 1 egg

- 30 ml. milk

- salt, pepper

COOKING:

Cut chicken into pieces. Mix it with frozen vegetables. Beat an egg with milk. Lay out vegetables and chicken on a baking sheet, cover this with beaten egg, add salt, pepper and bake it for about 40 minutes at 200 C. You can add onions and cheese on top as well.

SKINNY PIZZA

Skinny pizza with mozzarella and turkey on the cauliflower base.

INGREDIENTS:

- 1/2 cauliflower

- 1 egg

- 200 g + 50 g nonfat mozzarella

- 2-3 tbsp. Parmesan cheese

- sea-salt

- fresh-ground black pepper

- 1/3 glass chopped tomatoes in own juice

- 2 tsp dried basil

- 2 tsp oregano

-1 glass cut cherry tomatoes

- 250 g turkey fillet

- 2 garlic calves

- 1/4 tsp paprika flakes

- 100 g light cheese (15% fat)

- fresh basil leaves

COOKING:

Preheat oven to 200 C. Grate cauliflower or crush it in the food processor. Place it in a big bowl and cook it in the microwave at the maximum power for about 7-8 minutes, or until soft. Take it out and cool down, if it is necessary, extract excess liquid. Beat an egg slightly and add 200 g mozzarella, parmesan, salt, freshly ground pepper and cauliflower. Carefully knead it by hand until smooth. Prepare baking paper. Lay out a base on the baking sheet, distribute it with fingers on all surface and bake it within 10-15 minutes or till it is golden-brown. Meanwhile fry the turkey fillet on the grill till golden-brown within several minutes, then chop it into small pieces. Cover cooked base for pizza with a sauce made of chopped tomatoes, then sprinkle dried basil and oregano. Lay out pieces of the remained mozzarella, turkey, cherry tomatoes, garlic and paprika, and sprinkle grated light cheese. Bake it until cheese melts, about 10-15 minutes. Decorate it with fresh basil before you serve it. Bon appetite!

MARINADE

How do you marinade chicken breast? I share my favorite super marinade for a moist chicken.

INGREDIENTS:

- 1-2 tsp apple vinegar (you can use balsamic vinegar)

- 1 tsp. mustard

- 1 tsp dried oregano or rosemary

- 2 grated garlic cloves

- 2 tbsp. olive oil

- spices

COOKING:

Put all ingredients in a plastic bag and shake it well. Add chicken breast to the same plastic bag and shake it once more to marinade equally. Leave it in the refrigerator for a couple of hours or overnight. When marinaded, bake it on the grill for 4 min. on both sides or in the oven at 180 C for 20 min.

CHICKEN BREAST WITH FETA CHEESE AND HERBS

CPFC in 100 g: 135/21/4.8/0.3

INGREDIENTS:

- 2 chicken fillet (1 full chicken breast)

- 150 g Feta cheese

- herbs (fennel, parsley)

- salt and black pepper

COOKING:

Cut a fillet in sticks (usually 6), add salt and pepper. Mix feta cheese with herbs. Spread this mixture on the chicken, roll them and roast for about 30-40 minutes at 180 C.

TANGERINE, BEETROOT AND TOMATO SALAD

INGREDIENTS (for 2 portions):

- 1 small beetroot

- 2 sweet tangerines

- 2 tomatoes

- 1 medium-size onion

- 100 g lettuce

- olive oil

- fresh ground black pepper

- wine vinegar

COOKING:

Peel and boil beetroot, cut it into cubes. Chop tangerines and peel its' skin. Cut tomatoes into cubes and chop lettuce. Mix all ingredients, add cut onion, largely cut pepper, salt, oil, and vinegar. Pepper has to be fresh-ground, so salad has that flavor.

AUTUMN SPINACH SALAD WITH PECANS

INGREDIENTS:

- 3 tbsp. olive oil

- 2 tbsp. apple vinegar

- 1 tbsp. mustard

- 1 tbsp. honey

- 1/2 tsp. sea-salt

- 1/4 tsp. black ground pepper

- 1 fine cut sour sweet apple

- 1/2 fine cut small red onion

- 2-3 cups spinach

- 1/2 glass raw pecan

COOKING:

Preheat a frying pan well on medium-heat. Put pecans on the pan and mix it often, so they don't burn. As soon as they begin to darken, remove them from fire and cool down. Mix olive oil, vinegar, mustard, honey, sea-salt and pepper in a small bowl until smooth. Put all ingredients in a big bowl; pour it with dressing and mix! Enjoy your meal!

TACOS WITH FISH

INGREDIENTS (for 8 portions):

- 3 cups shred cabbage

- ½ glass cut in cubes red onion

- 1 glass sour cream

- 1 rich lime

- ¼ tsp. salt

- 4 tilapia fillet

- ¼ tsp. paprika powder

- ½ tsp. dried garlic

- ½ tsp. cumin

- ½ tsp. salt

- ½ tsp. black ground pepper

- corn tacos (tortillas)

FOR SERVING:

- cilantro

- lime

COOKING:

Mix cabbage, red onion, sour cream, lime juice and salt in a big bowl. Put it in the refrigerator. Mix paprika powder, dried garlic, cumin, salt and black ground pepper in another bowl. Grease each tilapia fillet on both sides with a mix of spices. Fry fillet on medium-heat within 8 minutes on both sides. Cut the fish into small pieces with a fork and knife. Put tacos on the plate. Put cabbage and fish on top. Sprinkle lime juice and decorate it with cilantro. Enjoy your meal!

CUTLETS STUFFED WITH CHEESE

INGREDIENTS:

- 100g low-fat cheese

- 800 g chicken/turkey fillet

-1 onion

-1 egg

- 2-3 tbsp. herbs

- salt, pepper

COOKING:

Blend a fillet meat. Add and blend onion. Add eggs, herbs, and spices. Mix all ingredients. Take a part of mincemeat and hide a cube of cheese in it. Fry all meatballs without oil on the non-stick frying pan. Fry on medium-heat on both sides until golden-brown. Then add water and stew on low-heat for 10 more min. Done! Bon appetite!

BUCKWHEAT WITH CHICKEN AND MUSHROOMS

CPFC in total dish (1 portion): 295/26/5/38

INGREDIENTS:

- 100 g boiled buckwheat

- 80g chicken fillet

- 100g girolles mushrooms (or another kind)

- 1/2 small onion

- herbs

- salt, pepper

COOKING:

Wash mushrooms. Cut onion into small pieces. Fry onion with or without oil depending on the type of your frying pan. Chop chicken fillet into small pieces and fry it on the frying pan. Add salt and pepper. At the end add boiled buckwheat and herbs. Put it on a plate. Put pieces of the chicken on top. Add sour cream on top. Done! Bon appetite.

DELICIOUS SOUP WITH BROCCOLI AND CHICKEN FILLET INGREDIENTS:

- 500 g chicken fillet

- 1 big carrot

- 1 onion

- 300 g broccoli

- 300 g green beans

- salt, spices, bay leaf

COOKING:

Cook chicken in boiling water. Then add carrot and onion. After 10 minutes add broccoli and green beans. Boil it for 10 more minutes. Add salt, pepper, bay leaves and your favorite spices. Cook all ingredients on low-heat. Boil it for about 5 more minutes.

EGGS EN COCOTTE

INGREDIENTS (for 2 portions):

- 12 quail eggs

- 2 champignons

- 1 tomato

- a few cauliflower florets

- 1 tsp. olive oil

- 2 tbsp. cream

- salt, pepper

COOKING:

Cocotte is a special baking dish with 2 handles, it can be small or average size. Cut vegetables and put it in cocottes. Pour 1 tbsp. of cream in every cocotte. Add 6 quail eggs in every cocotte. Add salt and pepper. Bake it for 15-20 minutes. Bon appetite!

QUICK SNACK

INGREDIENTS:

- Low-fat cheese

- burrito bread

- 3 eggs

- cream cheese (low fat)

- chicken fillet (beat off and chopped)

- salt, pepper

COOKING:

Add salt, pepper to the beaten egg. Roll chicken fillet in this egg mix and then grill it for 1-2 minutes. Fry 2 eggs, keep yolk liquid. Grease burrito with cream cheese, strew it with grated cheese and lay out an egg on cheese. Lay chopped chicken fillet on the burrito. Add some more cheese on top, roll burrito and grill it for 20-30 seconds. Bon appetite!

CREAMY SALMON SOUP

CPFC in100 g: 124/12.6/4.2/9.5

INGREDIENTS:

- 400 g salmon

- 3-4 sweet potatoes

- cream cheese

- 1 onion

- 1 carrot

- salt, pepper, bay leaf

- herbs

COOKING:

Wash salmon and put it in a saucepan, add salt and cook until done (approx. 20-25 min). Cook onion and carrot in a frying pan until golden brown. When fish is cooked, take it out and separate meat from bones. Throw sweet potatoes cubes into a broth. After 15 min. add grated cream cheese (freeze it first and then grate). At the end, put the fish fillet back in the broth, add pepper and bay leaf. Boil it for 3-5 min., add herbs and leave it with no heat for 15 mins. Done!

CREAM OF PUMPKIN SOUP

INGREDIENTS (for 4 portions):

CPFC in 100 g: 39/5/1/4

- 1 chicken fillet (about 200 g)

- 400 g pumpkin

- 1 onion

- 50 g hard low-fat cheese

- salt, pepper, nutmeg

COOKING:

Wrap pumpkin in foil and bake it in a preheated to 180 C oven for 30 minutes. At this time cook chicken breast. Cut chicken into small pieces. Cut onions separately. Grate cheese. When the pumpkin is baked, cut it into large pieces, throw it into a broth and boil it within 5-7 minutes. Then add onions and cook another 5-7 minutes.

Add grated cheese, mix it well, add chicken and salt. Now use the blender to turn the soup into a puree. Enjoy!

OMELETTE WITH BROCCOLI AND BRIE CHEESE

- 400 g frozen broccoli

- 3 eggs

- 100 ml. milk

- 100 g brie cheese

- salt, pepper

- ground nutmeg and cardamom

- 2-3 fennel branches

- coconut oil

COOKING:

Steam broccoli. Grate cheese. Beat eggs in a bowl, add milk, spices. Add cheese and fine cut fennel to egg mixture. Mix it once again. Oil a casserole and layout broccoli in it. Cover broccoli with egg and cheese mixture. Bake in the preheated to 220C oven for 30 min. Serve it with favorite vegetables!

CHICKEN FILLET WITH CHEESE

INGREDIENTS:

- 2 chicken fillet

- 2-3 tomatoes

- 1 tbsp sour cream

- 70 g hard cheese

- 70 g Feta cheese

- fresh or dried basil

COOKING:

Cut chicken fillet in half, beat it, add salt, pepper, and grease with sour cream. Put tomato circles on top. Cut hard cheese in cubes (or grate). Crumble cheese feta by hand. Mix and spread on top of tomatoes, add fine cut basil. Put it in a fire-resistant baking dish and bake it for 30-40 min. Tasty and moist meat is ready!

SHAKSHUKA WITH HOME-MADE HUMMUS AND FRESH PITA BREAD

INGREDIENTS FOR HUMMUS:

- cooked chickpeas (300 g – dry chickpeas)

- 60 g tahini (sauce from sesame paste, lemon, garlic, water, and salt)

- 2 tbsp. lemon juice

- 2-3 tbsp. olive oil

- 3-4 garlic cloves

- salt, pepper

COOKING:

Mix all ingredients, except olive oil. Blend them using a blender. Add oil and continue to blend it until smooth. Keep it in the refrigerator in a closed container.

INGREDIENTS FOR SHAKSHUKA (for 2 portions):

- 1-2 red onions

- 4-5 garlic cloves

- 2-3 green peppers

- 3-4 medium-sized tomatoes

COOKING:

Stew all ingredients all together until soft. Serve shakshuka with fresh hummus and pita bread.

FISH CUTLETS

INGREDIENTS:

- 2 big white fish

- 1 onion

- salt/pepper

- semolina or whole grain flour

COOKING:

Wash and dry fish. Remove skin and bones. Grind it with 1 onion, add salt and pepper. Roll it in semolina (or whole grain flour) and form cutlets (8 pieces). Fry them in a non-stick frying pan. They may be a little bit watery but don't worry. Add nothing and wait until water evaporates. Keep frying them after this for about 3-4 more minutes on each side.

RICE NOODLES WITH VEGETABLES

INGREDIENTS:

- 1 package of frozen vegetables

- 2 portions of noodles

- sesame oil

- soya sauce, coriander, sesame seeds

COOKING:

De-freeze and stew vegetables, at the same time, boil noodles. Combine it in a frying pan, add sesame oil and soy sauce. Before serving, sprinkle it with sesame seeds and coriander.

DELICIOUS HARD BREAD

FOR DOUGH:

- 1 egg

- 80 g cottage cheese 2% fat

- 10 ml. milk

- 11 tbsp. oat flour

FOR FILLING:

- smoked meat/ham

- cheese

- multicolor tomatoes

- herbs

- olives

- sesame seeds

COOKING:

Mix ingredients for dough (it is better to blend it, it will be smooth). Put it in the refrigerator for about 2 hours or overnight! Cut meat, cheese, and tomatoes in cubes, cut olives in circles. Roll out dough on a silicone mat, average thickness, then lay out filling on it, wrap edges and sprinkle it with sesame seeds! Bake it in the preheated to 220 C oven for 30 minutes! Cool it down a little and enjoy the taste! Bon appetite!

SALMON AND VEGETABLES

INGREDIENTS:

- asparagus

- sweet potato

- zucchini

- salmon

- olive / another oil

- 1 garlic clove

- spices (salt, black powdered pepper, rosemary)

COOKING:

Preheat an oven to 200 C. Lay out asparagus, chopped sweet potato, chopped zucchini on the baking dish. Oil vegetables slightly, add salt, pepper, and garlic. Roast it for 15 minutes at 180-200 C. Lay out salmon over vegetables, add salt, pepper, rosemary and spray lemon juice. Roast it until fish is cooked (about 20-25 minutes).

APPLE PIE ENERGY BITES

INGREDIENTS:

1 glass of almonds

1/2 glass pecan nuts

1/2 glass dates

85 g dried apples

1/3 glass raisins

1/4 teaspoon ground cinnamon

1/4 teaspoon lemon zest

1/8 teaspoon sea-salt

COOKING:

Blend almonds and pecan nuts. Take out mixture out of the blender. Then blend dates, dried apples, raisins, lemon zest, cinnamon, and sea-salt. Add the mixture of nuts there and blend it all together once again. Form small balls of the received mixture and put it in the refrigerator for 30 minutes. Enjoy!

BLUEBERRY MUFFIN MUG CAKE

INGREDIENTS:

- 3 tbsp. fresh blueberry

- ¼ glass oat flour

- ½ teaspoon baking powder

- 2 tbsp. honey

- 1 egg white

- ½ teaspoon ground nutmeg

- Greek yogurt for serving

COOKING:

Mix an egg white and honey in the oiled mug. Add oat flour, baking powder, ground nutmeg and mix it well. Add fresh blueberries. Put it in the microwave on high power for 90 seconds (time can vary). Serve with Greek yogurt. Enjoy!

DARK CHOCOLATE BANANA BREAD

INGREDIENTS (for 10 slices):

- 3 ripe bananas

- 2 eggs

- ½ glass Greek yogurt

- ⅓ glass maple syrup

- 1 teaspoon vanilla

- 1 glass whole wheat flour

- baking powder

- ½ glass dark chocolate bars

COOKING:

Preheat an oven to 170 C. Mash bananas with a fork in a big bowl. Add eggs and mix it thoroughly. Add the rest of the liquid ingredients: Greek yogurt, maple syrup, and vanilla. Add flour, baking powder and mix it well. Melt chocolate pieces in the microwave. Add 1 glass of banana dough to a bowl with the melted chocolate and mix it well. Spread banana dough and then chocolate dough on top. Mix doughs with a knife or spoon accurately to make it look cool. Bake it for 40-45 minutes or until done. Cool it down for at least 15 minutes. Enjoy!

PROTEIN SMOOTHIE BOWL

INGREDIENTS (for 1 portion):

- 3/4 glass of frozen blueberry

- 1/2 frozen banana

- 1/3 glass oatmeal

- 1 tbsp. protein

- 1 tbsp. chia seeds

- 1 tbsp. lemon juice

- 1/3 glass almond milk

- 3 ice-cubes

FOR SERVING (not necessary):

- 2 tbsp. Greek yoghurt

- 1/2 kiwi

- 1 tbsp. cut almonds

- 1 tbsp. frozen bilberry

- 1 tbsp. goji berries

COOKING:

Blend blueberries, banana, oatmeal, protein, chia seeds, lemon juice, almond milk, and ice until smooth. Pour in a smoothie in a bowl, add Greek yogurt. Add kiwi, almonds, blueberries and goji berries on the top. Enjoy!

GINGER OATMEAL COOKIES

INGREDIENTS (for 8 cookies):

- 25 ml. honey

- 25 ml. Melted oil

- 1/4 teaspoon cinnamon

- juice of half lemon

- juice of half orange

- 10 g ginger root

- 100 g oat flakes

- 50 g almond flour

- 25 g sunflower seeds

- 25 g walnuts

- 20 g raisins

COOKING:

Grate small ginger and some lemon zest. Put it in a pan, add cinnamon, honey, lemon and orange juice. Heat it on fire without bringing to boiling temperature. Meanwhile, grind walnuts and raisins. Add flour, oat flakes and sunflower seeds. Mix it well. Mix liquid ingredients with dry. Add sunflower oil. Mix it and form cookies. Bake them for about 15 minutes at 180C till brown. Before serving, cool them down and dry up cookies. Bon appetite!

HEALTHY BLUEBERRY CRUMBLE

INGREDIENTS (for 4-6 portions):

- 3 glass of blueberries

FOR CRUMBLE:

- 1 glass oatmeal

- ½ glass almond flakes

- ¼ glass whole wheat flour

- ½ teaspoon cinnamon

- 2 tbsp. melted coconut oil

- ¼ glass maple syrup

FOR SERVING:

- ¼ glass Greek yogurt

- 2 tbsp. maple syrup

COOKING:

Preheat an oven to 180 C. Mix dry ingredients for a crumble in a bowl. Add liquid ingredients and mix it well. Spread blueberries in a medium-sized baking dish, spread crumble on top. Bake it for 45-50 minutes till brown. Mix Greek yogurt with maple syrup. Pour it in the crumble. Serve and enjoy!

TOASTED QUINOA, DRIED FIG & DARK CHOCOLATE GRANOLA BARS

INGREDIENTS:

- 1/2 glass oatmeal

- 1/2 glass quinoa

- 1/4 glass sunflower seeds

- 1/4 glass pumpkin seeds

- 1/2 glass organic sunflower oil

- 1/3 glass honey

- 1 teaspoon vanilla

- 1/2 teaspoon cinnamon

- 1/4 teaspoon sea-salt

- 1/4 glass flax seeds

- 1 tbsp. chia seeds

- 1/2 glass cut into large pieces dried fig

- 1 tbsp. chopped dark chocolate

COOKING:

Preheat an oven to 160 C. Distribute oatmeal, quinoa, sunflower seeds, and pumpkin seeds on a baking sheet equally. Bake it for 8-10 minutes. Pour it into a bowl and take it away. Mix sunflower oil, honey, vanilla, cinnamon and sea salt in a saucepan on low-heat until smooth. Remove it from fire and cool it down for several minutes. Add it to a bowl with oatmeal and quinoa. Mix it well. Add flax seeds, dried fruit and chia seeds. Cover baking sheet with a baking paper. Spread mixture and distribute it equally, press it strongly. Melt chocolate and pour on a granola bar. Put the baking dish in the freezer for 30 minutes or until mixture hardens. Take it out and cut it into 10 bars. Keep it in the refrigerator. Enjoy your meal!

TASTY MANGO MOUSSE!

INGREDIENTS:

- 2 teaspoon instant gelatin

- mango

- maple syrup

- 200 ml. Cream 10-20% fat

COOKING:

Prepare gelatin in water according to the instruction. Peel and grate mango. Add it to gelatin. Add 200 ml. of cream and a sweetener (syrup). Blend it until smooth. Pour it into baking cups and freeze it for 30 minutes or in the refrigerator overnight. Decorate it if you like. To reduce calories you can experiment with soft cottage cheese instead of cream.

BLUEBERRY BREAKFAST COOKIES (GLUTEN-FREE)

INGREDIENTS (for 8 pcs.):
- 2 tbsp. melted coconut oil
- 1/4 glass coconut sugar
- 1 mashed with fork medium-sized banana
- 1/2 teaspoon vanilla extract
- 1/2 teaspoon almond extract
- 1/4 glass flax meal
- 1/2 glass almond flour
- 1/2 teaspoon soda
- 1/2 teaspoon cinnamon
- 1/4 teaspoon salt
- 1 and 1/4 glass oatmeal
- 1 tbsp. chia seeds
- 1/2 glass frozen or fresh blueberries
- 1/4 glass chopped walnuts
- 55 g cut into large pieces dark chocolate

COOKING:

Preheat an oven to 175 C. Cover a baking sheet with a baking paper. Mix melted coconut oil, coconut sugar, banana puree, vanilla and almond extract in a big bowl until smooth. Add flax meal, almond flour, soda, cinnamon, salt and mix it before stiff dough formation. Add oatmeal, chia seeds and mix it accurately. At last add blueberries, walnuts, dark chocolate and mix it again accurately. Form cookies and bake it for 15-20 minutes until edges become slightly golden-brown. Cool down it for 15 minutes and enjoy!

SUPER CHOCOLATE GRANOLA

INGREDIENTS:

- 3 glass oatmeal

- 1,5 glass cut almond

- ¾ glass coconut flakes

- ½ glass cacao

- ¼ teaspoon salt

- ⅔ glass melted coconut oil

- ⅓ glass maple syrup (you can also use artificial sweetener or honey)

- 1 teaspoon vanilla

- 1,5 glass chopped dark chocolate

- sea-salt

COOKING:

Mix all ingredients. Created mixture you should spread on a baking dish evenly. Bake it in a preheated 125C oven for 50 minutes. Cool